Longer-Term Psychiatric Inpatient Care for Adolescents

Philip Hazell
Editor

Longer-Term Psychiatric Inpatient Care for Adolescents

A Multidisciplinary Treatment Approach

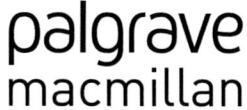

Editor
Philip Hazell
Walker Unit
Concord Centre for Mental Health
Concord, NSW, Australia

The University of Sydney
Sydney, NSW, Australia

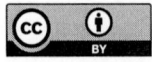

ISBN 978-981-19-1949-7   ISBN 978-981-19-1950-3   (eBook)
https://doi.org/10.1007/978-981-19-1950-3

This Palgrave Macmillan imprint is published by the registered company Springer Nature Singapore Pte Ltd.
The registered company address is: 152 Beach Road, #21-01/04 Gateway East, Singapore 189721, Singapore

Contents

v

Note on Contributors

Jaileen Alonzo is a registered nurse who has worked at the Walker Unit since 2017.

Kia Currell is a senior dietician at the Concord Centre for Mental Health. She trained at The University of Sydney and has worked across adult and adolescent mental health in both inpatient and outpatient settings. She has an interest in managing disordered eating behaviours in the context of existing mental illness.

Ariel Diaz is a clinical nurse specialist at the Walker Unit, with a particular interest in sport and physical wellbeing.

Meng Du is a registered nurse who has worked at the Walker Unit for several years.

Isabelle Feijo is a consultant child and adolescent psychiatrist and Unit Director. She trained in Switzerland before relocating to Australia. She has a special interest in family systems therapy.

Jacky Hanh is a clinical pharmacist with the Concord Centre for Mental Health. Hanh has a special interest in psychopharmacology and management of adverse drug reactions.

Philip Hazell is Conjoint Professor of Child and Adolescent Psychiatry at The University of Sydney, School of Medicine and a consultant child and adolescent psychiatrist with the Sydney Local Health District. In former roles as director of child and adolescent mental health services for the Hunter and Sydney Local Health Districts respectively, he was responsible for the commissioning of two psychiatric inpatient units for adolescents. Owing to this experience, he was called as an expert witness to the Barrett Adolescent Centre Commission of Inquiry, Queensland 2015-2016. Philip's current research focuses on adolescent development, the longitudinal course of disorders such as attention-deficit/hyperactivity disorder and bipolar disorder, and treatments for autism, deliberate self-harm and depression. He has 152 peer reviewed publications, 27 invited book chapters, and one monograph to his credit. From 2012 to 2014, he served as the Head of the Discipline of Psychiatry for The University of Sydney. For the Royal Australian and New Zealand College of Psychiatrists, he served on the Examinations Committee for six years, followed by six years as the Chair of the Subcommittee for Advanced Training in Child and Adolescent Psychiatry. He was recently the College nominee on a committee overseeing revisions to child and adolescent psychiatry training in New South Wales.

Steve Hoare is a Clinical Nurse Consultant. He trained in child and adolescent mental health nursing in the UK before relocating to Australia.

Stephen Ho is a the Nursing Unit Manager of the Walker Unit.

Kelly Jones is a certified practising speech pathologist. She works in adolescent and adult mental health settings and feels strongly that these services should meet the communication needs of the individuals who use them.

Tharushi Kaluarachchi is a clinical psychologist registrar. She completed an M.Clin.Psych at the University of Technology, Sydney. She has a special interest in creatively engaging adolescents in therapy using both verbal and non-verbal components.

Beth Kotze is a consultant child and adolescent psychiatrist, medical administrator and Director of Child and Adolescent Mental Health Services. She has worked in senior management and executive level positions for over 25 years, including at the central policy level for the Ministry of Health.

Polly Kwan is a senior occupational therapist. She trained at The University of Sydney and has a special interest in using sensory approaches and non-verbal therapy.

Bianca Lino is a clinical psychologist. She completed her M.Clin.Psych at The University of NSW and has a special interest in working with adolescents with major mental illness.

Nina Mather is a social worker who has worked in Human Services for 20 years, her specialty being Adolescent Mental Health. She holds qualifications in Single Session Thinking and Therapeutic Life Story work, and is a facilitator for various programs, such as "Tuning into Teens" and "Teen Got It".

Joanne McIntyre is a registered music therapist and has a Master of Creative Music Therapy as well as a B.Ed (Mus) and L.T.C.L. from The Trinity College of London. McIntyre has a particular interest working with young people and their identity through music.

Matt Modini is a clinical psychologist. He completed his PhD with The University of Sydney. He has a special interest in mental health inpatient treatment.

Fran Nielsen is a doctoral candidate and sessional academic at Western Sydney University and has forty years of experience in community arts and health projects. She has worked as an art therapist at the Walker Unit since it opened in 2009.

Kahlia Pollock is a registered nurse. She began working at the Walker Unit in 2017 and has since completed a Graduate Certificate in Applied Mental Health Studies (Child and Adolescent).

Mark Rawlinson is a registered nurse who began working at the Walker Unit soon after it opened.

Karen Sarmiento is a senior social worker and family therapist. She trained at Western Sydney University, the University of New South Wales NSW, and the Institute of Child and Adolescent Psychoanalytic Psychotherapy. Alongside systemic work, she has a special interest in child & adolescent psychoanalytic psychotherapy, in particular, the intrapsychic and intersubjective elements affecting illness, engagement and recovery.

Amanda Scali is the Assistant Principal of the Rivendell School. She completed her teacher training in Sydney at Macquarie University, majoring in History and English. She has worked in Special Education for 10 years.

Jennifer Shumack is the Principal of the Rivendell School.

ABBREVIATIONS

ACSQHC	Australian Commission on Safety and Quality in Health Care
ADHD	Attention-Deficit Hyperactivity Disorder
ADL	Activity of Daily Living
APAC	Australian Psychology Accreditation Council
ASD	Autism Spectrum Disorder
BPMH	Best Possible Medication Histories
CAMH	Child and Adolescent Mental Health
CAMHS	Child and Adolescent Mental Health Services
CBT	Cognitive Behavioural Therapy
CCMH	Concord Centre for Mental Health
CEC	Clinical Excellence Commission
CNC	Clinical Nurse Consultant
CNS	Clinical Nurse Specialist
COVID	Coronavirus Disease
DBT	Dialectical Behaviour Therapy
ECT	Electroconvulsive Therapy
EEG	Electroencephalogram
EMT	Emergency Management Team
ERP	Exposure and Response Prevention
IMP	Individual Management Plan
LHD	Local Health District
MDT	Multidisciplinary Team
MET	Medical Emergency Team
MOH	Ministry of Health
MRI	Magnetic Resonance Imaging
MRP	Medication Related Problem
NSW	New South Wales

NUM	Nursing Unit Manager
ODD	Oppositional Defiant Disorder
PDSA	Plan, Do, Study, Act
PLP	Personalised Learning Plan
PRN	Pro re Nata (as Needed)
QUM	Quality Use of Medicine
RANZCP	Royal Australian and New Zealand College of Psychiatrists
RMT	Registered Music Therapist
RN	Registered Nurse
RoSA	Record of School Achievement
SLSO	School Learning Support Officer
SNs	Specialty Networks
SSP	School for Specific Purposes
TAFE	Technical and Further Education

LIST OF FIGURES

LIST OF TABLES

LIST OF BOXES

CHAPTER 1

Introduction

Philip Hazell

Abstract The purpose of this book is to describe the multidisciplinary model of care delivered by a long stay high severity psychiatric unit for adolescents. We acknowledge that many jurisdictions do not have the resources to establish a unit that fulfils such a specialized role within the system of mental health care. Nevertheless, we hope that the learnings derived from the unit may generalize to other specialist adolescent mental health inpatient settings.

Keywords Adolescent • Inpatients • Mental disorders • Length of stay • Patient care team

Mental disorders are the most prevalent illnesses in adolescence and have the potential to carry the greatest burden of illness (WHO, 2014) and stigma into adult life. Governments in higher income countries have responded to this challenge by allocating more resources for

P. Hazell (✉)
Walker Unit, Concord Centre for Mental Health, Concord, NSW, Australia

The University of Sydney, Sydney, NSW, Australia
e-mail: Philip.Hazell@health.nsw.gov.au

© The Author(s) 2022
P. Hazell (ed.), *Longer-Term Psychiatric Inpatient Care for Adolescents*, https://doi.org/10.1007/978-981-19-1950-3_1

community-based and inpatient mental health treatment services directed to youth (Health Service Executive (Ireland), 2012; House of Commons Health Committee, 2014; National Mental Health Development Unit, 2009; NSW Health, 2011; Royal College of Psychiatrists, 2015). However, options remain limited for those young people with severe mental illness requiring secure inpatient care. Specialist child and adolescent mental health (CAMH) inpatient units are typically designed to provide short-term care when the acute phase of a mental illness poses danger to the young person or the community. The aims are to assess and to stabilize the young person then discharge them to treatment in the community. Length of stay is usually measured in weeks rather than months (Hazell et al., 2016). Unfortunately, some young people experience either repeated or unremitting episodes of mental illness requiring longer periods of inpatient treatment. Delivering such treatment in an acute mental health unit is feasible, but it requires the diversion of already limited resources to develop a customized treatment plan in an environment that is not fit for purpose (Thompson et al., 2021). In addition, repeated exposure to newly admitted, acutely unwell patients, can destabilize young people with chronic mental illness. Owing to the limited number of specialist acute CAMH beds, a proportion of young people experiencing chronic or relapsing mental disorders are redirected to adult mental health inpatient facilities (Hazell et al., 2016; Wheatley et al., 2004). In recognition of this problem the Ministry of Health for the state of New South Wales (NSW), Australia in a draft planning document stated

> To improve care for young people with significant impairment who require treatment in an inpatient setting due to continuing risk, two new additional specialist non-acute inpatient units will be established with state-wide roles and appropriate design and staffing arrangements for those who are still receiving involuntary treatment. NSW does not currently have specialised units of this type for young people. Care pathways to and from these units will be carefully considered and the allocations will need to factor access to families/carers and other community supports with appropriate accommodation options for visitors. (referenced in NSW Health, 2011)

Funding for the first of these units was announced in 2007, to be situated on the campus of a newly opened psychiatric hospital, and in close proximity to other CAMH services and a general hospital. After a planning phase of approximately 18 months, the unit opened in 2009. The purpose of this book is to describe the multidisciplinary model of care delivered by the unit. We acknowledge that many jurisdictions do not have the resources to establish a unit that fulfils such a specialized role within the system of care. Nevertheless, we hope that the learnings derived from the unit may generalize to other specialist CAMH inpatient settings. We are also mindful that longer stay inpatient care runs counter to the trend towards briefer hospital admissions within the context of a continuum of care (Blanz & Schmidt, 2000). We share the view that most young people experiencing mental health problems can be managed by community resources, augmented if necessary by brief admissions for crisis resolution. We do question how helpful such crisis admissions are, since the capacity to deliver therapeutic intervention is limited. For new patients such admissions may afford the clinical team time to arrange comprehensive community support. For a patient with a chronic or relapsing psychiatric condition this is no longer relevant. There is, as argued above, a subgroup of young people with serious mental disorders for whom a longer hospitalization is the optimal care.

The Walker Unit (named for nineteenth century NSW colonial politician, merchant banker and philanthropist Thomas Walker) was thus established as a specialist longer-term adolescent inpatient unit as part of the "phase of illness model of care" at the Concord Centre for Mental Health (CCMH). The "phase of illness model" delineates patient groups in order to target phase-specific treatments to improve patient outcomes. The Walker Unit is one of seven phase-specific mental health units at CCMH. Indications for the psychiatric hospitalization of children and adolescents include the need for intensive observation or investigation to inform diagnosis, to manage significant risk associated with a psychiatric condition or its treatment, or to manage medical complications of a psychiatric condition (Perkes et al., 2019). It was anticipated the reason for admission to the Walker Unit would mostly involve the management of risk arising from one or more of the following:

1. severe and unremitting psychotic disorders
2. severe and unremitting mood disorders
3. unremitting suicidality and dangerous deliberate self-harm
4. behavioural disturbance arising from neuropsychiatric conditions such as autism

Chronic and unremitting eating disorder was also considered, but lack of sufficient medical support especially for children under the age of 16 has precluded the admission of patients who are physically compromised. In addition, treatment for severe eating disorder is available from state-wide specialized inpatient units for adults and for young people operating from other hospitals in NSW. Young people with a history of criminal behaviour may be admitted to the Walker Unit, but there is a statewide juvenile forensic mental health inpatient facility operating from another location. Admission to the Walker Unit has, however, been used as a step-down from forensic hospital and to facilitate progressive re-integration to the community.

Most patients admitted to the Walker Unit have had a substantial period of treatment in an acute inpatient setting. Some patients are received through inter-hospital transfer, while others are admitted during a time when they are living in the community. Most have a high level of risk of self-harm and/or harm to others. A history of prolonged school disengagement or school dysfunction is a feature common to most young people attending the programme. Many also experience a family history of mental illness and/or chronic dysfunction and interpersonal difficulties, which have served to precipitate and/or exacerbate the severity and persistence of the mental illness and associated problems. While it was anticipated most patients would be detained under the provisions of the NSW Mental Health Act, the experience of the unit during the period 2015 to 2020 was that this was the case for only a minority (28%). The five most common primary diagnoses in the period 2015–2020 were depression (37%), schizophrenia (16%), post-traumatic stress disorder (12%), autism (7%) and obsessive-compulsive disorder (7%). We are aware that using the primary diagnosis to describe a patient population has its limitations. We examined data from structured diagnostic interviews conducted on a sub-group of patients admitted in the period 2020–2021. When all concurrent diagnoses were considered, the most common psychopathologies were anxiety (27%), depression (23%), non-schizophrenic psychosis (10%) attention-deficit/hyperactivity disorder (10%) and oppositional defiant disorder (10%). The second set of diagnoses more accurately reflects the day to day work of the Walker Unit.

Treatment at the Walker Unit includes multimodal strategies. The longer length of admission at the Walker Unit enables pharmacotherapy to be carefully reviewed and optimized. Most young people are prescribed less psychotropic medication on discharge than at admission. The psychotherapeutic treatments include evidence-based and novel interventions delivered via individualized, group-based and family-based formats to assist in the development and recovery of the young person. Weekly family therapy is designed to promote the lasting change required within the family system in order to help the young person maintain their mental health post discharge. An admission to the Walker Unit involves several phases encompassing assessment, the establishment of a therapeutic alliance, defining therapeutic goals, implementation of treatment strategies, and finally, planning transfer of care to facilitate re-integration into community-based treatment. Education programmes delivered by the Walker Unit Learning Centre provide essential components of rehabilitation and restoration of developmental tasks.

The short to medium term goal of the Walker programme is a reduction or remission in the presenting symptoms. The longer term goal is to achieve a level of independent functioning in the young person that is consistent with their mental age. Coexisting physical conditions requiring medical monitoring or support are managed through consultation with the relevant subspecialty unit of the adjacent general hospital, or in some instances with the nearest paediatric hospital. All young people are discharged to stable accommodation, but in some cases not to the care of their families. All young people have an established educational or vocational pathway on discharge, although this may not be a return to the previous school of enrolment. The experience of the unit has been that young people who have a mental illness severe enough to require intensive longer stay inpatient treatment typically need the support of a special needs school or program.

The Walker Unit endeavours to tailor its programme to meet the particular needs of the young person. In the early phases of an admission, most young people reside in the unit seven days a week. As the admission progresses, patients are granted increasing amounts of leave off the ward including overnight leave, used as part of re-integration to home and education. Although length of stay varies, in the period 2015 to 2020, goals were achieved within six months for 64% of patients. Admissions extended beyond a year for 6% of patients owing to exceptional circumstances. Long admissions were avoided where possible because of the risk of institutionalization and disengagement with resources in the community.

In the chapters that follow, we will examine the physical environment of the unit, and the adaptations that have been made to ensure its functionality. We will consider the therapeutic milieu and the role played by multidisciplinary team members individually and collectively in its maintenance. We will describe clinical processes such as admission and discharge planning, formulation and case review. We will consider the specific roles of professionals including nurses, teachers, psychotherapists, psychologists, social workers, art therapists, music therapists, speech therapists, occupational therapists, dieticians, pharmacists and medical staff. We will describe the suite of therapies offered to patients. We will describe the steps taken to maintain and enhance the physical wellbeing of patients, including the optimization of pharmacotherapy. We will describe how the unit operates within the framework of the Mental Health Act. We will consider training and education. Finally, we will describe how the unit responded to challenges caused by the COVID-19 pandemic.

Acknowledgement Parisa Fani-Molky (medical student, The University of Sydney) assisted in the preparation of this chapter by retrieving descriptive data and standardized measures from the electronic medical records.

References

Blanz, B., & Schmidt, M. H. (2000). Preconditions and outcome of inpatient treatment in child and adolescent psychiatry. *Journal of Child Psychology and Psychiatry, 41*(6), 703–712.

Hazell, P., Sprague, T., & Sharpe, J. (2016). Psychiatric hospital treatment of children and adolescents in New South Wales, Australia: 12-year trends. *BJPsych Open, 2*(1), 1–5. https://doi.org/10.1192/bjpo.bp.115.000794

Health Service Executive (Ireland). (2012). *Fourth annual child and adolescent mental health service report 2011–2012.* http://www.hse.ie/eng/services/Publications/services/Mentalhealth/camhs20112012annualreport.pdf.

House of Commons Health Committee. (2014). *Children and adolescent's mental health and CAMHS. Third report of session 2014–2015* (Vol. 2015). House of Commons.

National Mental Health Development Unit. (2009). *Working together to provide age-appropriate environments and services for mental health patients aged under 18.* A briefing for commissioners of adult mental health services and child and adolescent mental health services. http://www.nmhdu.org.uk/silo/files/publication-working-together-to-provide-ageappropriate-environments-and-sces-.pdf

NSW Health. (2011). *Children and Adolescents with Mental Health Problems Requiring Inpatient Care.* PD2011_016. NSW Health.

Perkes, I. E., Birmaher, B., & Hazell, P. L. (2019). Indications for psychiatric hospitalization of children and adolescents. *The Australian and New Zealand Journal of Psychiatry, 53*(8), 729–731. https://doi.org/10.1177/0004867419835930

Royal College of Psychiatrists. (2015). *Faculty report CAP/01: Survey of in-patient admissions for children and young people with mental health problems.* Royal College of Psychiatrists.

Thompson, A., Simmons, S., & Wolff, J. (2021). Nowhere to go: Providing quality Services for Children with Extended Hospitalizations on acute inpatient psychiatric units. *Journal of the American Academy of Child and Adolescent Psychiatry, 60*(3), 329–331. https://doi.org/10.1016/j.jaac.2020.09.009

Wheatley, M., Waine, J., Spence, K., & Hollin, C. R. (2004). Characteristics of 80 adolescents referred for secure inpatient care. *Clinical Psychology and Psychotherapy, 11*(2), 83–89.

WHO. (2014). *Health for the World's adolescents. A second chance in the second decade.*

CHAPTER 2

The Physical Environment

Stephen Ho and Steve Hoare

Abstract Many readers will have worked in facilities that were once state-of-the-art in design, but have become unfit for the purpose. Capacity to modify the physical environment of a psychiatric unit in response to changing clinical need or practice is essential. The Walker Unit differs from adolescent units at other locations because of its larger internal footprint and greater secure outdoor space. Substantive modifications to the Walker Unit over time have included requisitioning of space to create a learning centre, modification of some bedrooms to create a parent retreat, the establishment of a sensory room, and repurposing of the seclusion area to become a de-escalation suite. The chapter will describe the physical environment of the Walker Unit referenced to Australasian Health Facility Guidelines, and current best practice.

Keywords Adolescent • Inpatients • Health facilities

S. Ho • S. Hoare (✉)
Walker Unit, Concord Centre for Mental Health, Concord, NSW, Australia
e-mail: Stephen.Ho@health.nsw.gov.au; Steve.Hoare@health.nsw.gov.au

© The Author(s) 2022

P. Hazell (ed.), *Longer-Term Psychiatric Inpatient Care for Adolescents*, https://doi.org/10.1007/978-981-19-1950-3_2

9

INTRODUCTION

The Australian Health Facility Guidelines stipulate that inpatient mental health units for young people require "a conscious balancing of the requirement to provide an effective therapeutic environment for acute mentally ill young people with the need to provide them and their families' visitors and staff with a pleasant, spacious light filled, comfortable and homely facility" (Australasian Health Infrastructure Alliance, 2016). Domestic style furnishings and décor should be homely not custodial, and in shared spaces should be movable to make adjustments for activities.

The environment should support the provision of safety and privacy of young people, allow for spaces where individual therapy can be conducted confidentially, group therapy and educational activities can be conducted for larger groups and recreational activities can be planned and undertaken. The environment should have capacity to offer smaller containing zones that can be used to separate young people experiencing distress, away from the wider patient group to prevent what Sergeant (2009) describes as the "Domino effect" where distress spreads among young people. These containing areas should enable distraction and sensory modulation activities to take place and reduce the noise created during distress from affecting the wider ward area. In situations where there is an event of behavioural disturbance such as aggression, the ability to move the wider group of patients to a different area where the programme can continue, reduces the need for physical restraint.

HISTORY

The public announcement that an adolescent unit would be established on the Concord Centre for Mental Health campus was made when the Centre was partially built (see Fig. 2.1). The ward allocated for this purpose was originally intended as an adult extended care unit. As such, considerable modification to the design was required from the outset to accommodate the needs of mentally unwell adolescents. Fortunately, some of these modifications were made while the original build was in progress. For example, the areas labelled "Arts and Crafts" and "Group Room" in Fig. 2.2 were redesigned to accommodate the Learning Centre, while the area labelled "Activities" became the Art Therapy space. Subsequent modifications have been made to respond to the need for structural improvement,

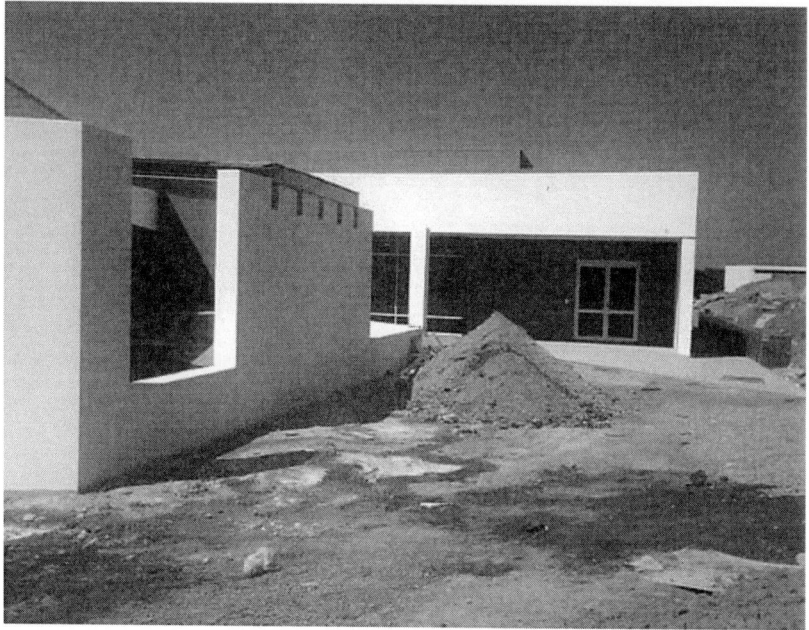

Fig. 2.1 Phase of build at the time the ward was repurposed from an adult extended stay unit to an adolescent high severity longer-stay unit

repurposing of space, privacy, infection control, and Occupational Health and Safety (OH&S) concerns.

The responsibility for facility planning first rested with the health district's Director of Child and Adolescent Mental Health Service (CAMHS), the nursing unit manager of an existing adjacent medium severity adolescent mental health unit, the principal of the school providing learning centre support to the unit, and the Mental Health Facility Planner. They worked from the floor plan illustrated in Fig. 2.2. The Director recalls the challenge of trying to imagine from the floor plan how the unit would look in real life, as 3-D imaging was not available to the team. After commissioning responsibility for facility planning, it was transferred to the unit's newly appointed nursing unit manager and psychiatrist director, supported by the CAMHS and Mental Health Service executives.

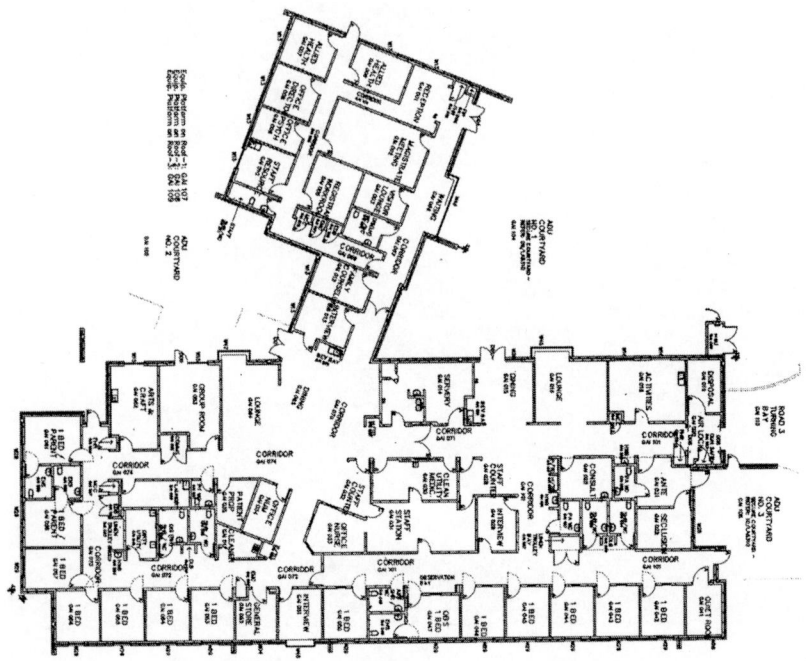

Fig. 2.2   The Walker Unit floor plan at the time of commissioning

MODIFICATIONS

Since the Walker Unit opened in 2009, there has been extensive modification to address clinical risks and to ensure that the environment is both therapeutic and safe. The original fit out of the building posed a number of safety hazards. For example, fire extinguishers were placed in common areas, where they could have been used by an assaultive patient as weapons. Bedrooms contained items that could be misappropriated for self-harm, such as exposed metal screws in the light fittings and metal strips under the doors. Once identified these hazards were removed and replaced.

As the clinical programme evolved, use of the available space within the unit changed. For example, the adoption of trauma informed care principles has altered greatly the way in which the seclusion area is used. Originally used for time out, and sometimes the emergency administration of medication, it now forms part of a suite of low stimulus options for young people who are emotionally and behaviourally not regulated.

A quality project as well as a needs analysis were conducted over a two year period from 2012–2014 incorporating physical environment, practices and policies through several Plan, Do, Study, Act (PDSA) cycles. An inventory and stocktake of what we had and what we required and wished for was discussed through several planning meetings. The design of several spaces such as the development of the parents retreat room and sensory spaces were envisaged and planned for future implementation.

Since the original building was completed, there have been a number of capital work adaptations:

1. Creation of a parent retreat room, including en-suite bathroom and overnight facilities such as a sofa-bed, within an accessible bedroom and en-suite.
2. Extending an interview room and creating a purpose built sensory room.
3. Changing a high secure bedroom into a quiet room and then into a staff resource room.
4. Adding secure doors to the main corridor and opening up two bedrooms to create the High acuity POD, which includes a bedroom, en-suite and living area that can be securely maintained as a containment area.
5. Creating a purpose built musical instrument store in the space where music therapy is undertaken.

Description of Current Ward Physical Environment

The Walker Unit is a large inpatient unit offering 11 bedrooms, 6 of which are located off a secure corridor, a number of lounge areas, three outdoor courtyards, a sensory room, art room and de-escalation suite all surrounding a central nursing office, secure kitchen and dining area. The unit contains a two-roomed Learning Centre, parent's retreat room, and two interview rooms. Managing risk and supporting safety is a key feature of the physical environment. Safety checks are undertaken by staff before young people enter the unit to ensure an environment free from items that can be used to cause harm. Delaney et al. (2018) describe inpatient CAMHS units as providing an "aseptic" environment free from fixtures and furnishings that can be used for the purpose of self-harm; some of the modifications made at the Walker Unit are depicted below (Figs. 2.3, 2.4

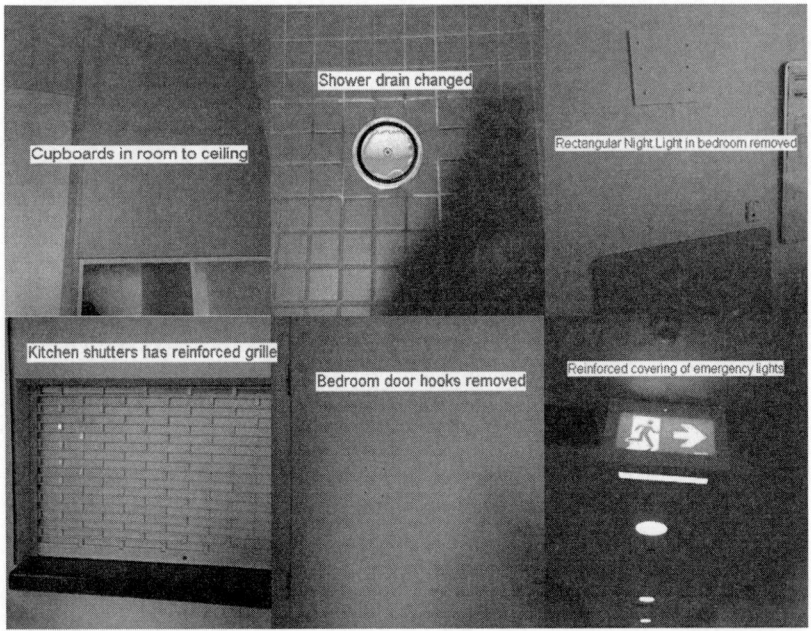

Fig. 2.3 Adaptations made to improve safety

and 2.5). All windows have thickened secure glass, all doors accessing the ward area have viewing windows to prevent young people absconding when doors open. A duress alarm system works throughout the unit spaces.

Separating Spaces

The Walker Unit was designed so that it could function as two separate zones. When a young person needed a more secure space to support their safety and privacy away from other young people, it was common practice to move either the young person or the wider group into the other zone. However, when the second side was used to support an individual, access to some facilities was compromised. In 2021, capital works were undertaken to create a "High acuity POD". This area can now be locked off from the rest of the unit, provide a living and dining space, bedroom and en-suite bathroom and securely contain a young person with lesser restrictions on space for the wider group. This POD space is located by the parent retreat room and has secure access to a courtyard. This space provides

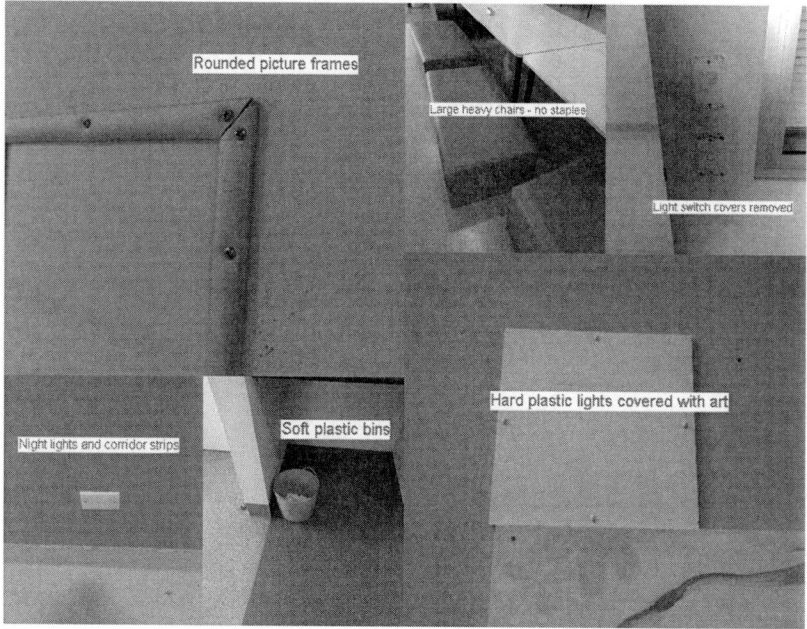

Fig. 2.4 Adaptations to improve safety

containment for acutely unwell young people on admission to the Walker Unit. When this space is not required for containment, it is kept open and offers a third lounge area and seating area that can be used to provide group or family therapy.

SINGLE BEDROOMS

Each young person has their own bedroom with shared single use bathrooms. Each bedroom contains a tamper-proof bed preventing a hiding place for contraband, fixed shelving, desk and bedside table and a magnetic locked cupboard. The bedrooms have blinds between the window panes so no curtains, which could provide ligature fixtures, are required. Six of the bedrooms are accessed via a secure corridor adjacent to the nursing station allowing for close observation. In the secure corridor, the bedroom doors are fitted with a window with integrated blinds that can be operated from the outside to enable regular checking on the young people's wellbeing. Bedrooms in the secure corridor can have their doors

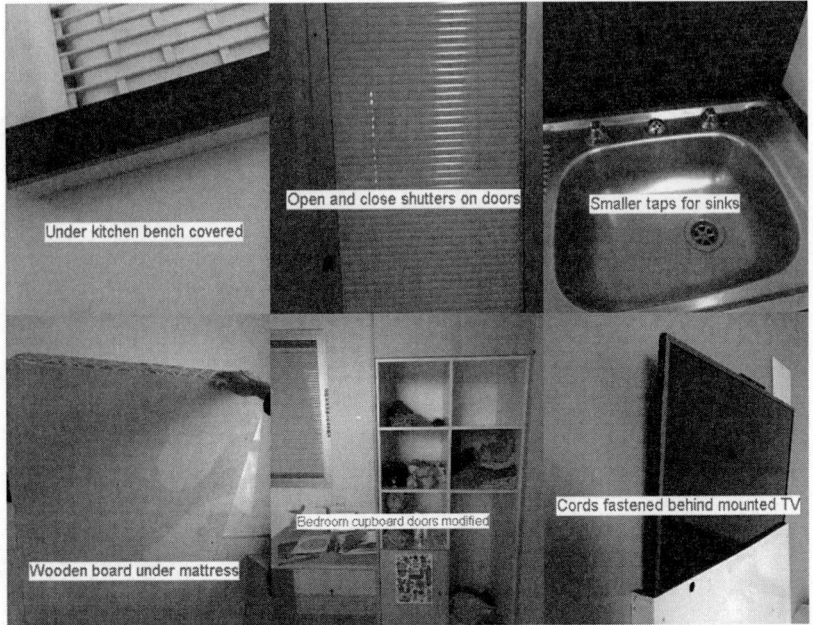

Fig. 2.5 Adaptations to improve safety

removed to prevent barricading by a young person who may attempt being unsafe. The use of single bedrooms and bathrooms allow for capacity to accommodate gender diverse young people without having to make obvious environmental adjustments, supporting both their needs and confidentiality. Young people are encouraged to bring in bedding and decorations from home to make their room feel homely and inviting. Bedrooms are locked during the hours of the therapy programme, but can be accessed on request as needed.

Multipurpose Spaces

The main lounge and dining area provides space for all young people and staff to eat meals, run group activities, hold community meetings and farewell events at discharge, and run school assemblies. It is within view of the nursing station. The other ward areas; interview rooms, art room, sensory room and de-escalation suite routinely are spaces used for individual therapy sessions, smaller family meetings or supporting individuals experiencing difficulties away from the busier area offering more privacy and reduced sensory stimulation.

Outdoor Spaces

There are three courtyards available at the Walker Unit, offering access to a trampoline, basketball rings, exercise bike, rowing machine and punching bag. One courtyard is specifically designed as a sensory garden, with musical instrument fixtures, artificial grass, water sprinklers, orange and lime trees and a sand pit (see Chap. 13). All the courtyards have modified designs that include anti-climb fencing and walls. Access to a courtyard is supervised by staff and duress sensors can detect alarms in these areas. As with the internal spaces, frequent environmental searches must take place in the courtyard to remove items that could be used to self-harm with such as broken glass or sharp objects. During the warmer months, each Friday lunch, the unit has a barbeque and all the staff and young people dine together outside.

Staff Presence and Availability

Engaging young people in meaningful activities, learning centre or programme activities, or relaxing and social recreational activities in the evening is central to being able to observe young people's behaviour and the dynamics amongst the wider group so as to provide support or intervention when required. In a large space such as the Walker Unit, the ability to plan activities with young people and manage the space, so that staff can observe and engage does include the ability to close the space down and open spaces in a planned way to account for the needs of the young people.

If We Knew Then What We Know Now

1. Outdoor space should be well maintained, plants and bushes trimmed to allow clear view underneath to prevent hiding of contraband items. Outdoor spaces should be well lit so they can be used in evenings when it becomes dark as a space to offer a variety of de-escalation activities.

2. Consider having spaces available that can be closed into more private, containing space, to be able to support young people in distress away from the wider unit population. Distressful noise can contribute to a cascade effect, disturbing other young people and triggering distress.
3. Have the capacity to close the wider areas of a unit down in the evening, as part of the night time routine and focus activities in fewer spaces.

CONCLUSION

The physical environment of an adolescent inpatient unit is a constantly changing one. Several modifications and improvements have been made to the Walker Unit to address risk and safety, which have necessitated in minor capital works and changing practices. The balance of being a therapeutic space versus safety and containment is always a challenge, however, just as young people learn from practical experience, so do the staff adapt with ongoing practical solutions.

REFERENCES

Australasian Health Infrastructure Alliance. (2016). *Australasian health facility guidelines. Part B- Health Facility Briefing and Planning*. 0132-Child and Adolescent Mental Health Unit.

Delaney, K. R. (2018). Nursing in child psychiatric milieus: What nurses di: An update. *Journal of Child & Adolescent Psychiatric Nursing, 2017*(30), 201–208. https://doi.org/10.111/jcap.12204

Sergeant, A. (2009). *Working within child and adolescent mental health inpatient services: A practitioners handbook*. Quality Network for inpatient CAMHS. U.K.

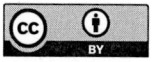

CHAPTER 3

The Milieu

Fran Nielsen, Ariel Diaz, Meng Du, Kahlia Pollock, Jaileen Alonzo, and Mark Rawlinson

Abstract Given the typical length of admission young people hospitalised at the Walker Unit may spend somewhere in the vicinity of 3–5% of their current lifespan living in the facility. It is imperative therefore that the admission affords the opportunity for engagement in a developmentally appropriate therapeutic programme, while at the same time maintaining safety. Patient mix, including phase of recovery, has an important impact on the ward milieu. Safety is maintained through observation and engagement. A level system the young people have helped design promotes and rewards skill development and prosocial behaviour. The chapter will describe the strategies the Walker Unit uses to maintain safety while at the same time addressing adolescent needs such as access to social media, interaction with peers, and sexual safety.

Keywords Adolescent • Inpatients • Aggression • Self-injurious behaviour • Atmosphere

F. Nielsen (✉) • A. Diaz • M. Du • K. Pollock • J. Alonzo • M. Rawlinson
Walker Unit, Concord Centre for Mental Health, Concord, NSW, Australia
e-mail: Fran.Nielsen@health.nsw.gov.au; Ariel.Diaz@health.nsw.gov.au; Meng.
Du@health.nsw.gov.au; Kahlia.Pollock@health.nsw.gov.au;
Jaileen.Alonzo@health.nsw.gov.au; Mark.Rawlinson@health.nsw.gov.au

P. Hazell (ed.), *Longer-Term Psychiatric Inpatient Care for Adolescents*, https://doi.org/10.1007/978-981-19-1950-3_3

Introduction

Central to the young person's experience on a mental health ward is the milieu. This can be an integral aspect of their recovery and to be successful a therapeutic milieu needs to maintain the safety of both patients and staff (Baeza et al., 2013; Creed et al., 2021; Thibeault et al., 2010). The policies and practices are formulated to maximise the possibility of creating a therapeutic milieu. In turn, the milieu can have an impact on the young person's behaviour and potential for recovery. One of our nurses has said, "An effective nursing environment has to have the capacity to 'hold' and guide the individual through the downs as well as identify the ups."

Background

Since the 1920's literature on the therapeutic milieu for child and adolescent mental health services has focused on how to manage difficult behaviours (Delaney, 2006; Petti, 2016). Safety, structure and support have been some of the key factors identified for a therapeutic milieu (Delaney, 1994, 2017; Petti, 2016). Recently there has been a move towards developmentally sensitive patient collaboration, embracing trauma informed care principles (DeSocio et al., 1997; Dotson, 2019). For children, adolescents and families with complex mental health histories planning for a 3–6 month length of stay can be helpful and this will also contribute to the milieu. For example, interactions with family, overnight leave and school integration are all considerations for the maintenance of a therapeutic milieu (Petti, 2016; Thomas et al., 2002). Progress in the peer group setting can also be assessed and further support discharge planning.

An important consideration in the development of the Walker Unit programme was the safe management of aggression. While everyone in the multi-disciplinary team is responsible for ensuring safe practice, the nursing staff have the most interactions with the young people and they are therefore central to maintaining the therapeutic milieu. Few of the nurses employed in the early years of the Walker Unit's operation had specific child and adolescent mental health experience. A number of the experienced nurses now working at the Walker Unit were recruited via a transition programme which introduced them to mental health nursing through a placement on the unit. While the newness of the Unit and the staff created tension in the milieu, it motivated the staff to seek training, especially with regard to the safe management of aggression. It coincided with a statewide initiative to reduce the use of restraint and seclusion in mental health facilities, which meant that training opportunities were abundant.

Staff continuity contributes to a therapeutic milieu (Petti, 2016) and the transition nurses that have returned to the Walker Unit after their training have had a positive impact on the development and implementation of non-reactive approaches. One nurse has reported, "if the team is feeling they can trust one another it will complement the whole ward dynamic, because you have a team that can work more confidently together. If there are unfamiliar staff that are not confident to sit with the level of distress in the young person this will impact the milieu, the patient can pick up on anxieties in staff."

To support therapeutic interactions in the milieu there is an organised educational and allied health programme throughout the day. Refer to Chap. 9 for more detail on this topic. Nursing staff support the young people's attendance within the timetabled programme and engage them with quiet activities in the evening.

DEVELOPMENTAL CONSIDERATIONS

Many of the patients are prone to unpredictable aggression which is more often manifested in unstructured time. Staff are required to engage young people creatively and genuinely, especially when there is less structure in place that is, afternoons/evenings and weekends when the group therapy programme is finished. Staff need to be mindful of each young person and their developmental needs by being proactive in their engagement. This means staying on the floor as much as possible and interacting either in a group or in an individual setting (Delaney, 1994; Petti, 2016). Their developmental age and intellectual capacities are variable and at times staff are required to sit with a young person's distress, ensuring they understand what is expected of them. It is during these times that as a team we need to be mindful of the impact a young person in distress has on the ward.

One of our nurses is quoted as saying, "it is important we work together and be available to one another, as well as engaging the other young people who are still present on the ward and who are impacted by their peer's distress." Teamwork within the nursing and wider team requires role modelling from senior members of the team as well as providing training opportunities for staff to assist with their development and further their skills. This is explored further in Chap. 6. Regarding developmental considerations and the lessons learned in creating a safe and therapeutic milieu for children, adolescents and their families DeSocio et al. (DeSocio et al., 1997) write, "A sense of humour and the ability to sidestep power struggles are useful tools in forming an alliance with the adolescent" (p. 24).

Patient Mix

Patient mix, which encompasses gender, maturity, severity of illness, nature of illness, and phase of recovery, has an important impact on the ward milieu. The Walker Unit team has found it better to have no more than two patients with emotionally dysregulated self-harm and/or aggressive behaviours at a time. Above this number, the other young people on the Unit tend to copy undesirable behaviours. They may collude with each other to bring in contraband (if one young person has leave with a lesser search on return/ if one young person has leave when others don't), or cause disruptions or major incidents on the ward. Young people with similar presentations and difficulties may also compete in self-harming behaviours or may cause distress among each other (contagion). The introduction of a new and typically unstable patient alters the dynamic between young people.

When nursing staff manage and support the new young person's distress/self-harm episode, it affects the rest of the young people in the unit. For example, one young person may get traumatised from witnessing incidents and this can trigger their past traumas, leading to increased thoughts of self-harm and at times act on them. Some may get over-involved and need gentle redirection to move away from the incident and allow staff to de-escalate.

It is not unusual for patients to have met each other during prior hospitalisations in one of the state's acute CAMHS inpatient units. The previous relationship history has the potential to influence ward dynamics. For example, two young people who may have a history of colluding on other wards, may continue this behaviour and disrupt the ward milieu, for example, suicide plans and group absconding.

A Collaborative Behavioural Intervention

Safety is maintained through observation and engagement. A level system the young people have helped to design promotes and rewards skill development and prosocial behaviour (see Chap. 6). The Walker Achievement Level System encompasses generalised expectations and privileges and customised expectations and privileges. These are reassessed in the weekly reviews with risks and safety concerns addressed daily. Token economies and level systems are often linked with developing a young person's self-awareness and in turn, a therapeutic milieu (Petti, 2016). For example, in this level system a young person might not be given access to their SIM card or the kitchen on the ward for safety reasons but may be encouraged to have leave with their family where they can practice this access safely at home. Another example of how this level system is utilised may be with an unmotivated young person, who would be encouraged to access the kitchen or individual short walks off the ward to challenge their anxieties and develop their independence. The further up in the level system the young person achieves, the more independence and competence with regard to safety they will have demonstrated. Maintaining a close eye on what motivates the young person can contribute to a healthy therapeutic milieu.

Safety Strategies

Addressing adolescent needs such as independence and safety with regard to social media and interaction with peers is a daily challenge on the ward. Thinking about sexual safety, verbal and physical aggression, bullying and self-esteem are common themes within the therapy programme on the ward. Some of these topics will be addressed in individual therapy, family meetings, group therapy and individual sessions with allied health, medical, and nursing staff. This contributes to stabilising the ward and building a therapeutic milieu. For example, if one young person is feeling isolated or attacked by their peers on the ward, staff will support collaborative activity to process the difficult feelings that are being experienced. There may be some non-verbal group therapies like music, art or sport in combination with psycho-education to bring the young people together safely first and then addressing the topic of bullying verbally as it arises. If the young person continues to feel isolated or attacked by peers this can be further explored in their individual therapies or discussions with nursing staff to work on strategies and plans for therapeutic change.

Staff burnout is also a safety concern, and this is supported by regular individual and group supervision for nursing staff. If this is not addressed, staff can become tired and reactive, contributing to poor clinical judgement with an increased risk for patients, for example, secluding a patient for a behaviour that posed minimal risk or the over-use of PRN medications. Some of the topics of concern identified by nursing staff and discussed in supervision include the traumatic histories these families bring to the admission, compassion fatigue and the vicarious impact of traumatic incidents such as suicide attempts and self-harm. Reflecting on the way we talk about the work has characterised how we manage the work and the therapeutic milieu. For more details on the topic of nursing supervision, refer to Chap. 6.

Supervision engenders confidence in staff to balance risk and containment with the principle of least restrictive practice. Examples might include staff supporting the parents to allow the young person to have unescorted leave or to travel back from school by public transport. Sometimes the parent's anxieties can have a greater impact on the ward milieu than the young person. Maintenance of the therapeutic milieu requires excellent communication between staff. When there are lapses in communication, chaos and stress can occur. For example, a parent might drop off a stressed young person after leave without a handover to staff, or staff may not open the courtyard for a young person to access the trampoline when it's in their care plan. When staff are not paying attention to the milieu, the young people will often respond with anxiety and destructive behaviour because they are feeling unsafe.

One of the safety-tools the nursing team have developed as a proactive intervention for some of the young people that struggle with their aggression, is the 'De-escalation tree' (see Fig. 3.1). In collaboration with the young person, nursing staff will clarify at each stage what the options are with the goal to reduce restraint and/or seclusion. The flow chart can be modified in consultation with the young person and this has contributed to their engagement towards a therapeutic milieu. This has been a helpful tool for regular nursing staff introducing unfamiliar nursing staff, as it clearly outlines and promotes a collaborative non-reactive thoughtful response to the young person's distress. Regular de-briefing with the young people using chain analysis will occur if the young person or staff member have had difficulties with working in the distress.

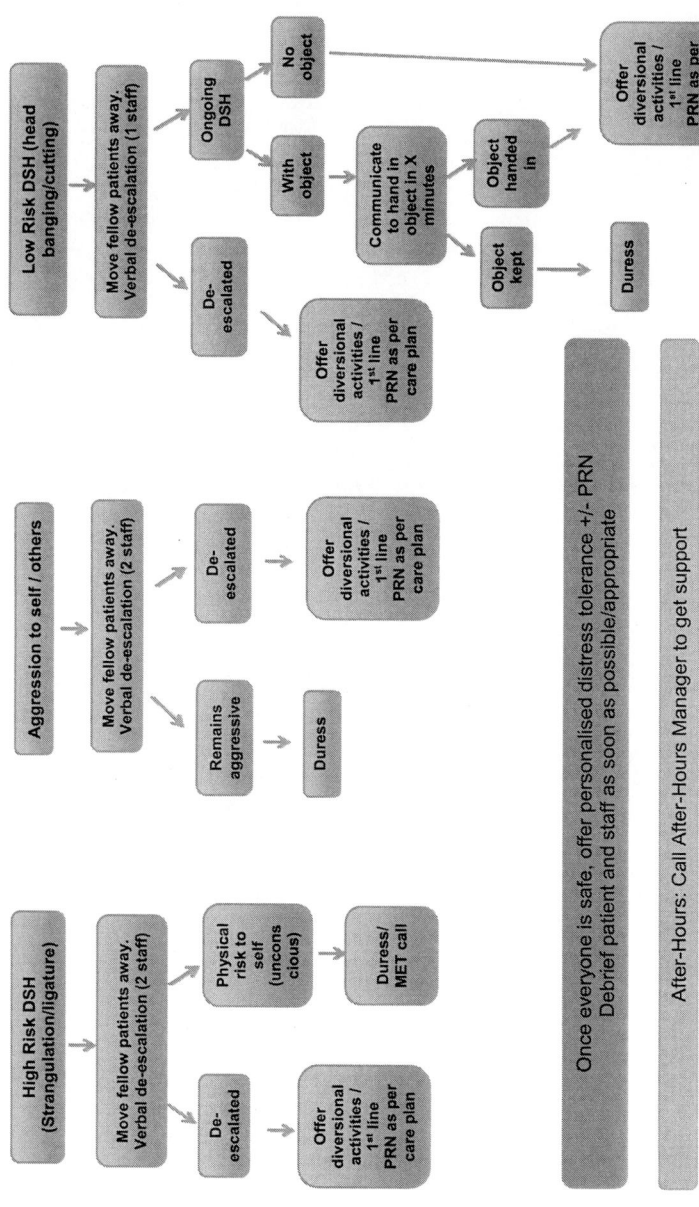

Fig. 3.1 De-escalation tree

REFERENCES

Baeza, I., Correll, C. U., Saito, E., Amanbekova, D., Ramani, M., Kapoor, S., Chekuri, R., De Hert, M., & Carbon, M. (2013). Frequency, characteristics and management of adolescent inpatient aggression. *Journal of Child and Adolescent Psychopharmacology, 23*(4), 271–281. https://doi.org/10.1089/cap.2012.0116

Creed, T., Waltman, S. H., & Williston, M. A. (2021). Establishing a collaborative care CBT milieu in adolescent inpatients units. *Cognitive Therapy and Research., 45,* 428–438. https://doi.org/10.1007/s10608-020-10134-z

Delaney, K. R. (1994). Calming an escalated psychiatric milieu. *Journal of Child and Adolescent Psychiatric Nursing, 7*(3), 5–13. https://doi.org/10.1111/j.1744-6171.1994.tb00199.x

Delaney, K. R. (2006). Top 10 milieu interventions for inpatient child/adolescent treatment. *Journal of Child and Adolescent Psychiatric Nursing, 19*(4), 203–214. https://doi.org/10.1111/j.1744-6171.2006.00072.x

Delaney, K. R. (2017). Nursing in child psychiatric milieus: What nurses do: An update. *Journal of Child and Adolescent Psychiatric Nursing, 30*(4), 201–208. https://doi.org/10.1111/jcap.12204

DeSocio, J., Bowllan, N., & Staschak, S. (1997). Lessons learned in creating a safe and therapeutic milieu for children, adolescents, and families: Developmental considerations. *Journal of Child and Adolescent Psychiatric Nursing, 10*(4), 18–26. https://doi.org/10.1111/j.1744-6171.1997.tb00418.x

Dotson, N. (2019). Facilitating the development of a patient empowered milieu: Moving from paternalism to patient collaboration in an acute adolescent inpatient psychiatric unit. *Journal of Child and Adolescent Psychiatric Nursing, 32*(3), 162–164. https://doi.org/10.1111/jcap.12249

Petti, T. (2016). Milieu treatment: Inpatient, partial hospitalization and residential programs. In M. K. Dulcan (Ed.), *Dulcan's textbook of child and adolescent psychiatry* (2nd ed., pp. 939–953). American Psychiatric Association Publishing.

Thibeault, C. A., Trudeau, K., d'Entremont, M., & Brown, T. (2010). Understanding the milieu experiences of patients on an acute inpatient psychiatric unit. *Archives of Psychiatric Nursing, 24*(4), 216–226. https://doi.org/10.1016/j.apnu.2009.07.002

Thomas, S. P., Shattell, M., & Martin, T. (2002). What's therapeutic about the therapeutic milieu? *Archives of Psychiatric Nursing, 16*(3), 99–107. https://doi.org/10.1053/apnu.2002.32945

Open Access This chapter is licensed under the terms of the Creative Commons Attribution 4.0 International License (http://creativecommons.org/licenses/by/4.0/), which permits use, sharing, adaptation, distribution and reproduction in any medium or format, as long as you give appropriate credit to the original author(s) and the source, provide a link to the Creative Commons licence and indicate if changes were made.

The images or other third party material in this chapter are included in the chapter's Creative Commons licence, unless indicated otherwise in a credit line to the material. If material is not included in the chapter's Creative Commons licence and your intended use is not permitted by statutory regulation or exceeds the permitted use, you will need to obtain permission directly from the copyright holder.

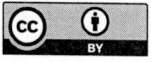

CHAPTER 4

Admission and Discharge Planning

Isabelle Feijo, Steve Hoare, and Karen Sarmiento

Abstract It is essential that staff of an adolescent inpatient psychiatry unit have the capacity and authority to ensure parents and treating community clinicians support the admission, families participate in the treatment, and community clinicians participate in discharge planning and assertive follow up since these are features known to improve clinical outcomes. The chapter outlines, through the use of a hypothetical case example, the processes involved in admission to and discharge from the Walker Unit.

Keywords Adolescent • Inpatients • Referral and consultation • Patient admission • Patient discharge

INTRODUCTION

The Walker Unit is part of a state-wide CAMHS continuum of care that includes centre based and mobile community based treatment teams, residential and day programs, acute adolescent mental health inpatient units, a young person's forensic unit and a rehabilitation and sub-acute unit. The

I. Feijo (✉) • S. Hoare • K. Sarmiento
Walker Unit, Concord Centre for Mental Health, Concord, NSW, Australia
e-mail: Isabelle.Feijo@health.nsw.gov.au; Steve.Hoare@health.nsw.gov.au;
Karen.Sarmiento@health.nsw.gov.au

© The Author(s) 2022
P. Hazell (ed.), *Longer-Term Psychiatric Inpatient Care for Adolescents*, https://doi.org/10.1007/978-981-19-1950-3_4

Walker Unit also interfaces with other mental health providers including general adult psychiatric services, specialized early psychosis teams, youth mental health services, and private practitioners.

THE ADMISSION JOURNEY

Referrals are triaged by senior members of the team. If a young person is likely to benefit from the program an assessment team visits them, their family, and current treating team at the hospital or community centre where the patient is treated with the aim to gather more information to assist with treatment planning in the case the young person is admitted to the Walker Unit. The second step in the admission process consists in inviting the young person and their family for a visit to the Walker Unit for further exploration of the suitability and the commitment to the program. Admission dates are spaced so the unit is only settling in one new patient at a time. The Walker Unit team works collaboratively with the referring agency, the young person, and the family in planning for discharge, finding appropriate accommodation, facilitating access to educational or occupational programs, and arranging treatment with local mental health services.

The following hypothetical case example illustrates the admission journey:

> At referral Monica was a 15 year old girl, the second of four siblings, living with her mother, mother's new partner, her three siblings and 3 year old half-brother in a regional location. Monica presented with recurring medically serious self-harm and unremitting suicidality in the context of dysphoric mood. Her diagnoses were complex post-traumatic-stress-disorder and probable borderline personality disorder. During her primary school years Monica was sexually molested by a neighbour. She was referred by the consultant psychiatrist of an acute adolescent psychiatric inpatient unit for consideration of a transfer to the Walker Unit. Transfer was requested because while self-harm had remitted during two previous hospitalisations, the behaviour had returned after discharge to the community. There was significant functional impairment. Monica had not consistently attended school during the previous two years. She was affiliating with an older delinquent peer group who facilitated substance abuse. In the community Monica had received cognitive behaviour therapy and dialectical behaviour therapy, but her engagement with treatment was indifferent. She had also received adequate trials of fluoxetine, sertraline, and venlafaxine, each augmented with quetiapine. For logistic reasons family therapy had not been attempted, but the parents were described as burned out by Monica's diffi-

culties, and two of her younger siblings were manifesting anxiety symptoms. The referrer sought a comprehensive diagnostic review.

Following the conversation between the consultant psychiatrists, the ward secretary sent a referral pack to Monica's current treating team. The contents of the pack are summarized in Box 4.1.

Once the completed referral pack was returned, senior Walker clinicians discussed the case during a weekly Intake meeting to determine if Monica could potentially benefit from an admission to the Walker Unit. One consideration was whether she was truly treatment resistant or if she was better characterised as treatment avoidant. The determination was that best endeavours had been employed to engage Monica in evidence-based psychological therapy in the community, and this had been supported by adequate trials of first and second-line pharmacotherapy. The Intake team decided to proceed to the next stage of admission planning, an assessment meeting undertaken at Monica's present location (regional acute inpatient unit). As per usual practice the assessment would be undertaken by a consultant psychiatrist, clinical nurse consultant, and an allied health professional.

Box 4.1 Walker Unit Referral Pack

To support the referral of {insert name} to the Walker Unit please provide the following information.

1. summary letter including formulation and goals of a Walker admission
2. risk assessment form
3. discharge summaries from inpatient admissions (including reports of investigations such as MRI, EEG, blood results, etc.)
4. incident reports during admissions
5. psychological therapy reports
6. family intervention reports
7. any cognitive, speech, language and occupational therapy assessments
8. education reports
9. nursing care plans and
10. reports of referrals to other agencies such as Child Welfare Services

In preparation for the assessment visit, the clinical nurse consultant contacted the referring team to request that the whole family (including all siblings) attend the meeting. The assessment team travelled to the hospital where Monica was admitted. The assessment team first met with the current treating team to receive an update on progress, to further clarify the objectives of a transfer to Walker, and to clarify any queries arising from the written referral material. They then met Monica and her family to assess motivation and capacity to engage in treatment. Monica expressed ambivalence stating, "What's the point. I'm going to kill myself when I turn 16 anyway" but also described longer-term educational and career goals. The team explored the family's understanding of Monica's difficulties, willingness to support an admission, and engage in regular family sessions. Information was provided about the ward program and the various therapeutic modalities described in other chapters of this book. Particular emphasis was given to the importance of family engagement. This is because experience has taught us that some parents, particularly those who have become burned out, see a Walker admission as primarily an opportunity for respite.

After the assessment meeting, the assessment team discussed the readiness of Monica and her family for an admission to the Walker Unit. Owing to the therapeutic intensity of the Walker treatment program considerations for admitting a young person must include a number of perspectives; the level of clinical dependency of the current cohort, such as supervision for activities of daily living or meal times, the cohort's capacity to engage in the program or providing individualised activities and the potential for risk behaviours and contagion between cohort members. The team believed Monica and her family were ready and motivated for an episode of care at the Walker Unit and recommended proceeding to the next stage of the admission assessment, a visit by Monica and her family to the ward.

The pre-admission visit afforded the family to ask any questions that had arisen from the first meeting. The team reaffirmed the family goals for an admission and their commitment and capacity to attend weekly family sessions. Monica and her family were given a booklet that outlines the program, including level system and expectations. The family were given a tour of the facility so that they may better understand the environment that Monica may be living in for six months or so. Monica and her family at this point agreed to an admission. In other circumstances, families have sought more time to consider their decision. An admission date was agreed on. Admissions are usually arranged for a Monday or Tuesday, so the patient can be settled in during a period of maximum staffing (Fig. 4.1).

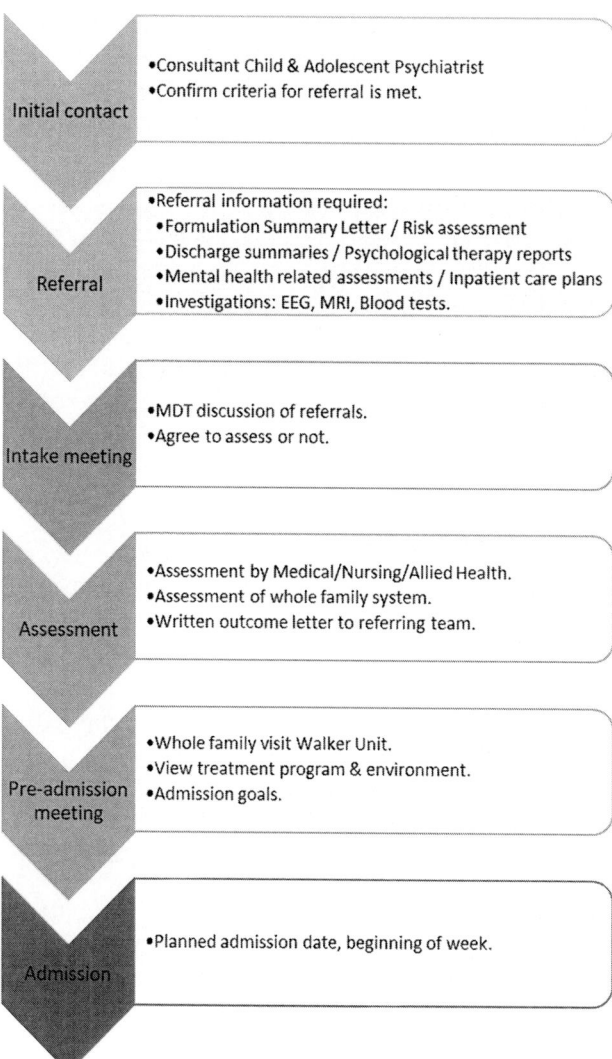

Initial contact
- Consultant Child & Adolescent Psychiatrist
- Confirm criteria for referral is met.

Referral
- Referral information required:
  - Formulation Summary Letter / Risk assessment
  - Discharge summaries / Psychological therapy reports
  - Mental health related assessments / Inpatient care plans
  - Investigations: EEG, MRI, Blood tests.

Intake meeting
- MDT discussion of referrals.
- Agree to assess or not.

Assessment
- Assessment by Medical/Nursing/Allied Health.
- Assessment of whole family system.
- Written outcome letter to referring team.

Pre-admission meeting
- Whole family visit Walker Unit.
- View treatment program & environment.
- Admission goals.

Admission
- Planned admission date, beginning of week.

Fig. 4.1 Assessment and pre-admission process

Prior to Monica's admission date the clinical nurse consultant identified the staff directly providing her treatment; primary nurse team, lead primary nurse, psychiatrist, registrar, individual therapist, family therapists, education team and any specific therapist such as a dietician or speech pathologist. To orient the treating team the clinical nurse consultant drew an admission summary diagram which includes the simplified genogram of the young person and their family; a summary of the presenting problem, diagnoses, number of past admissions, illness characteristics; summary of risks in admission; list of medications; summary of educational history; aims of admission from the individual and family system perspective and suggested care plans required to support the young person and the list of the team (see Fig. 4.2). This summary diagram was emailed to all team members, discussed in the morning report meeting before Monica arrived and displayed in the nursing office the week prior to admission.

The assessment team reviewed Monica's risk history both within hospital and in the community and made recommendations for her care. It was determined that Monica could be managed in the general ward rather than requiring an initial period in the high acuity POD area (see Chap. 2).

Preparation for Discharge

Discharge planning is part of the admission planning process and is considered during the multidisciplinary team formulation and review meetings (see Chap. 5) and the weekly care planning meetings. Identification of discharge location, educational pathway, and support services are prioritised from the start of the admission as these can have implications on the length of stay. The discharge destination may be different to the living arrangement prior to the admission depending on the circumstances of the young person's mental illness, the capacity of the families to support the needs of the young person and to maintain the safety of the young person and others. Discharge home is preferred, but alternatives such as at a different family member's home, supported accommodation, out of home care supported by child welfare services or alternative mental health facilities for those with continuing treatment needs (such as e.g., a young person with treatment resistant schizophrenia). For the majority of young people, attendance at a mainstream school is not possible and an access request is made for a place in a School for Specific Purposes (SSP) which typically has higher support levels for students. The process of allocating places in SSPs is done only once per school term by the Department of Education. As such, the possibility of an SSP referral has to be made early in the course of hospitalisation at the Walker Unit so that, if successful, there is adequate time to integrate the patient to the new school setting (see Chap. 7).

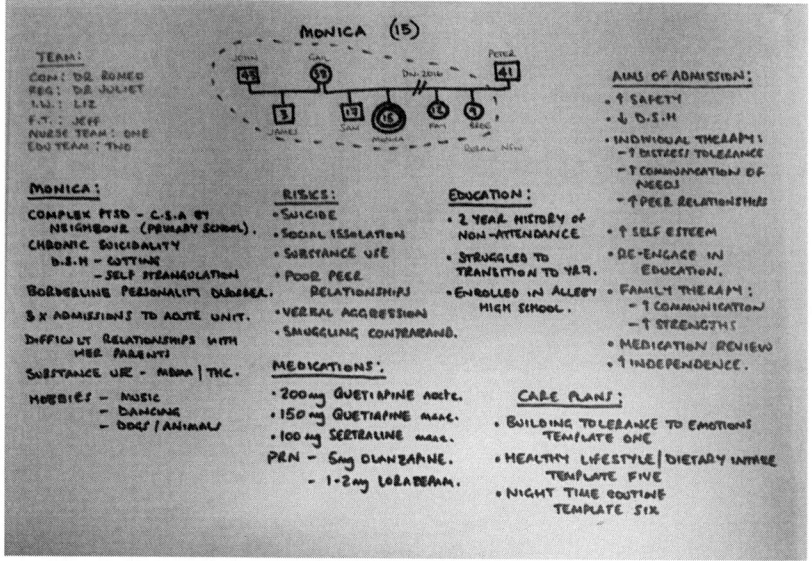

Fig. 4.2 Summary diagram of admission information

Practicing leave at their discharge location, being integrated into school and re-engaging the community support staff who will receive transfer of care back after discharge all form part of the treatment process and transition out of the Walker Unit. Graduated exposure to home and community settings is typically undertaken on weekends, and when a young person returns to the unit reviewing leave periods and understanding challenges and successes is done in family meetings. Problem solving difficulties experienced during leave forms part of continuous planning for the next leave period.

The community team is invited to the final MDT formulation and Care Planning in person or via video conference to be updated on the progress and changes during the admission and to discuss the follow up after discharge. We encourage community teams to visit the young person at home, at their home school, or at the Walker unit ahead of discharge. It is not uncommon for young people who are nearing 18 to be transitioned from the Walker Unit to an adult mental health team or service. In these circumstances, initiating the introductions of case managers to young people is attempted.

The discharge from the Walker Unit involves a farewell event for all young people and their families. The key team members provide a review of the admission and reflect on achievements and changes that have occurred during the admission for the young person and also for the family. The teaching team highlights the learning goals that were reached and awards that were distributed. The treating team also acknowledges the potential challenges ahead post discharge but highlight also the strengths they have shown during their admission. The young person and their parents have then an opportunity to reflect and comment on their experience of the admission.

The Walker team provide a seven day follow up call to all young people and their families to support the transition back to the community. This call offers families and young people to share any concerns or challenges they are experiencing with a familiar clinician, who can support problem solving, or connect with community clinicians and support their needs going forward.

It is not uncommon for former patients and families to make contact with the unit, not only during the initial months following discharge, but also to share milestone experiences such as starting a university course, passing their driving licence, or getting a job. In the event that contact is made with staff, there is a logbook for staff to complete, documenting the details of the contact and its nature. If there is any concern raised during contact such as deteriorating mental health or safety concerns, a staff member will liaise with the discharge community team to ensure that information is shared.

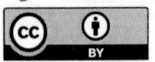

CHAPTER 5

Formulation and Case Review

Philip Hazell

Abstract A formulation integrates information derived about a patient to inform diagnosis and management. Cases referred to the Walker Unit are complex, and are likely to have been reformulated many times in the light of new information, and in response to evolution in the clinical problem. After a period of observation, assessment and investigation, the multidisciplinary team develops a formulation using a Five P structure, and identifies the patient's strengths and vulnerabilities. The process informs the development of a management plan which is presented to the patient and family for comment and endorsement. The process is repeated at six to eight weekly intervals throughout the admission. In addition, weekly case review meetings occur to examine progress against treatment goals, and to fine tune the management plan.

Keywords Adolescent psychiatry • Protective factors • Prognosis • Social environment

P. Hazell (✉)
Walker Unit, Concord Centre for Mental Health, Concord, NSW, Australia

The University of Sydney, Sydney, NSW, Australia
e-mail: Philip.Hazell@health.nsw.gov.au

© The Author(s) 2022
P. Hazell (ed.), *Longer-Term Psychiatric Inpatient Care for Adolescents*, https://doi.org/10.1007/978-981-19-1950-3_5

BACKGROUND

The formulation is a set of explanatory hypotheses or speculations that link the findings from the history (obtained from multiple sources), mental state examination, family assessment and investigation. According to guidelines prepared by the Royal Australian and New Zealand College of Psychiatrists (RANZCP) the formulation addresses the question: 'Why does this patient suffer from this (these) problem(s) at this point in time?' (Royal Australian and New Zealand College of Psychiatrists, 2012). As such, the formulation is a living document that will be modified as new information comes to light. Two common models for organising the formulation in child and adolescent mental health are the biopsychosocial formulation and the Four Ps (Henderson & Martin, 2014). As the name suggests, the biopsychosocial formulation organises information into biological, psychological and social domains. The model is intended to encourage holistic thinking, rather than attributing a child's problem to a single cause. Examples of the latter are attributing depression solely to an inherited predisposition to neurotransmitter dysfunction (biological), or anxiety solely to the experience of bully victimisation (social). The Four Ps model is a more sophisticated extension of the biopsychosocial formulation that allows consideration of chronology and aetiology, and suggests targets for intervention. The model considers predisposing, precipitating, perpetuating, and protective factors (Henderson & Martin, 2014). Variations of the model include statements about the presentation, pattern and prognosis (Nurcombe, 2014). In some versions there is a statement about management (Royal Australian and New Zealand College of Psychiatrists, 2012).

FORMULATION AS APPLIED AT THE WALKER UNIT

The Walker Unit team uses an adaptation of the Four P model which adds a statement about the presentation (see Table 5.1). We are mindful that formulation in child and adolescent psychiatry must take into account the developmental trajectory of the child, and consider the possibility that problems may be evolving rather than fixed. The *presentation* covers relevant signs and symptoms as well as pertinent negatives (i.e., key absent symptoms). We also consider incongruencies, that is, features that do not seem to fit with the overall pattern of symptoms. An example is a 14 year old boy who appeared to have major depression, but was needing to sleep

Table 5.1 Example of a care plan

Clare MRN XXXXX03
1st Care Plan - 4 August 2021
Page 1

Issues problems	Discussion/intervention	Staff
Genogram Boat Builder June 2018 December 2018 19 17 15 G H F C K D		
Strengths/achievements – Motivated to change – Friendly – Polite	– Respecting boundaries – Less oversharing	Clare
Psychiatric Diagnosis – Persistent depressive disorder – Posttraumatic stress disorder	– Complete structured diagnostic interview	Psychiatrist
Presenting – Emotional dysregulation – Interpersonal difficulties – Escalating self-harm – Complex posttraumatic stress disorder		
Medications – Fluoxetine – Prazosin – Melatonin – Quetiapine - as needed	– Consider switch to a more sedating antidepressant to replace fluoxetine, prazosin and melatonin	Psychiatrist/ psychiatrist in training
Predisposing – Wilm's tumour in early childhood and its treatment – Family history mood disorder, substance abuse		
Risks – Sexual safety – Interpersonal conflict – Medical complications of Wilm's tumour treatment	– Monitoring	Team

(continued)

Table 5.1 (continued)

Clare MRN XXXXX03 1st Care Plan - 4 August 2021 Page 1	Issues problems	Discussion/intervention	Staff
Precipitating – Parent discord and separation – Sibling mental illness – Sexual safety incidents in and out of hospital – Changing parent roles	Sensory/living skills – Independent in activities of daily living	– No action required	
Perpetuating – Challenges to treatment engagement – Family communication – Estrangement from mother	Individual therapy – Dislikes pauses and silence in verbal – Cannot tolerate full session – Tolerates silence in visual modality	– Speak to previous therapists – Structured approach—Cognitive Behaviour Therapy – Individual art therapy	Psychiatrist in training Art therapist
Protective – Parent support for treatment – Evidence of resilience	Family therapy – H absent from sessions – Unresolved feelings about Wilm's tumour	– Engage H – Session with father's new partner, G	Clin psychologist/psychiatrist

Clare MRN XXXXX03
1st Care Plan - 4 August 2021
Page 2

Group therapy – Engages well in groups – Tests boundaries	– Maintain boundaries	Team .../2
School – Capable at year level – Gaps in knowledge owing to missed time	– Liaise with home school	Learning centre staff
Physical health – No known residual problems from neoplasia Plan/discharge/follow-up – EstimatedDateofDischarge:- Friday, 4 Nov 2021	– Obtain paediatric oncology records	Psychiatrist in training
Goals – Improved interpersonal relations – Engagement with school	– Negotiate other family goals	Clin psychologist/Psychiatrist

Signatures
Doctor
Patient
Parent/Guardian

as soon as he returned home from school. An MRI investigation revealed he had a pituitary adenoma. Family dysfunction is a dominant *predisposing* factor in most cases admitted to the Walker Unit (see the case example below). *Precipitants* may be discrete and obvious, such as exposure to a traumatic event. More typically, precipitants are diffuse events that have multiple impacts. Examples include the separation of parents, or the transition from primary school to high school. Sometimes it is not clear cut if something is a precipitant, or part of the presenting problem. An example might be ingestion of high potency cannabis followed by a psychotic episode. Is the drug use simply a trigger for the psychosis, or is it part of the presenting problem (e.g., an attempt at self-medication, or part of a more extensive substance use disorder?). Given the chronicity of the problems experienced by young people admitted to the Walker Unit, there are almost always *perpetuating* factors. Addressing them is an essential component of our therapeutic work. An example is a 17 year old girl who repeatedly sabotaged her treatment in the community through non adherence and disengagement. After a promising period of improvement in response to new treatment, the same pattern recurred during hospitalisation. Family work identified that although the parents were legally separated, there was blurring of boundaries between households and generations, and ambiguous communication between the parents. Family therapy promoted clearer communication between the parents, and a better delineation of household and generational boundaries. The patient was then able to engage productively in her own psychotherapy and art therapy, and accepted and responded to pharmacotherapy. *Protective* factors reduce the impact of stressors and symptoms, and promote recovery. Examples include personal attributes or skills, or features in the social environment such as a supportive school. Protective factors may be conspicuously absent in patients referred to the Walker Unit. We endeavour to be genuine rather than tokenistic in describing protective factors, as it is not helpful to say things simply to 'be nice'.

We anticipate that by the time a young person reaches the Walker Unit there will have been multiple formulations. Indeed, we ask the referring child and adolescent psychiatrist to provide a formulation which, ideally, should make clear the indications for a longer stay high severity admission. The Walker Unit team allow themselves about three weeks to undertake observation and targeted assessment before attempting a reformulation. It is presented during the first of what will typically be several meetings of the clinicians directly involved in the young person's care (the Mini Team) that occur during the course of hospitalisation.

Example of a formulation:

> Clare is a 15 year old female presenting with repeated self-harm, non-organic abdominal pain, low distress tolerance, oppositionality, low mood, hypervigilance and sleep problems. Her difficulties occur in the context of estrangement from her mother, peer problems, and school disengagement. The problems began around the onset of puberty. Predisposing factors are genetic vulnerability (as evidenced by mental illness in Clare's mother and brother), a tendency to adopt the sick role (stemming from the experience of Wilm's tumour in early childhood), impulsivity and rejection sensitivity. The diagnosis of Wilm's tumour and its treatment had a profound impact on the family. Clare's mother was for a long time disengaged from Clare's two elder siblings. The elder sister responded by adopting a pseudo parental role, while the brother became anxious and, eventually, depressed. Following Clare's recovery her mother slipped into depression and substance misuse. The parents had a conflicted separation. Perpetuating factors are the breakdown of parental authority, carer burnout, and the splitting and fragmentation of treatment services. In addition, multiple hospitalisations in crisis have led Clare to become experienced in the role of a mental health patient. Protective factors are the low lethality of the self-harm, and the observation that Clare is both resourceful and articulate. Despite their differences both parents are committed to Clare's treatment and recovery. The presentation suggests complex post-traumatic stress disorder or personality disorder. A major mood disorder is less likely. Residual cognitive deficits arising from chemotherapy need to be ruled out.

At the first Mini Team meeting the formulation is placed in a template alongside columns for issues/problems and discussion/intervention on a whiteboard. From this process flows a set of actions. The whiteboard work is transcribed to a word document and presented to the young person and their family for discussion and consent (see Table 5.1). As such the language used needs to be 'consumer friendly'. We do not, however, suppress content that may be confronting to family members. In Clare's case, for example, we were explicit about mother's substance misuse. The Care Plan is the road map for clinical care. It highlights matters that require intervention, but also indicates where the patient is already functioning adequately. In Clare's case for example, unlike many of the patients on the unit at the time she was fully independent with her self-care.

CASE REVIEW

The multidisciplinary team meets weekly to review the progress of all current inpatients. The group is much larger than the Mini Team and includes medical and allied heath staff, Learning Centre staff, peer support worker, at least one nursing team member, and the pharmacist. As such it is labour intensive, and therefore must be run efficiently. The meeting is chaired by the Unit Director and follows an agreed structure (see Box 5.1). Ten minutes is allocated to each case.

Box 5.1 Format of Case Review for Each Patient

1. Nursing report
2. Learning Centre report
3. Individual therapies
4. Family therapy
5. Group therapies, including peer support
6. Physical health and medication
7. Achievement level and leave considerations

Staff are encouraged to be structured and succinct in their reports. Discussion is welcomed, provided it is focused on the interests of the patient. The Chair needs to be vigilant and respond to dynamics that can derail the case review process. Examples include:

1. A staff member uses the presentation as a forum to debrief about their interaction with the patient or family. The Chair will encourage the staff member to take the issue outside of Case Review and discuss informally, or in supervision.
2. The case discussion uncovers some inconsistencies or errors in ward policy and procedure. The Chair will redirect these matters to the monthly staff meeting.
3. The case discussion uncovers splitting in the staff. The chair will redirect the matter to bi-weekly external supervision.
4. Strong opinions are expressed in the absence of information. The Chair encourages participants to follow clinical process and first gather sufficient information.

A successful case review will monitor progress against treatment goals, and fine tune the management strategies that have been outlined in the Case Plan. Examples of the latter could include adding individual art therapy for a young person who experiences difficulty verbalising emotions in talking therapy, or engaging the occupational therapist to provide training on public transport use to a young person who will need to travel by train to their new school of enrolment after discharge. Profound changes in management, such as an amendment to the discharge destination, are typically reserved for the more in-depth Mini Team reviews. Mini Team reviews also provide the forum for the clinician completed rating scales mandated by the state health authority. These are; Health of the Nation Outcome Scale for Children and Adolescents, Clinical Global Assessment Scale, and Factors Influencing Health Status.

Conclusion

Formulations and case review promote a team consistent approach with the aim to be containing for the family and the young person during their journey at the Walker Unit. The formulation changes over the admission and the family as a whole learn to adopt a broader (non-linear) thinking which takes the focus away from the identified patient. By coming up with evolving care plans and asking the patients to contribute to the weekly case reviews the young person is encouraged to advocate for themselves and learn to problem solve. It is not unusual that towards the end of an admission families and patients have adopted this way of thinking and during extended leave periods they are able to manage difficulties without the assistance of professionals.

References

Henderson, S. W., & Martin, A. (2014). Case formulation and integration of information in child and adolescent mental health. In J. M. Rey & A. Martin (Eds.), JM Reys's IACAPAP e-textbook of child and adolescent mental health: International associaton for child and adolescent psychiatry and allied professions. https://iacapap.org/content/uploads/A.10-CASE-FORMULATION-2014.pdf

Nurcombe, B. (2014). Diagnosis and treatment planning in child and adolescent mental health problems. In J. M. Rey & A. Martin (Eds.), JM Reys's IACAPAP e-textbook of child and adolescent mental health: Internatonal association for child and adolescent psychiatry and allied professionals. https://iacapap.org/content/uploads/A.11-TREATMENT-PLAN-2014-1.pdf.

Royal Australian and New Zealand College of Psychiatrists. (2012). 2012 fellowship program observed clinical activity (OCA) formulation guidelines. https://www.ranzcp.org/files/prefellowship/2012-fellowship-program/oca-formulation-guidelines.aspx

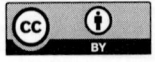

CHAPTER 6

Nursing Care

Steve Hoare and Stephen Ho

Abstract Of all professional groups, the nurses at the Walker Unit have, undoubtedly, the greatest contact with patients. Much of this contact is informal, through supervision of activities of daily living and unstructured time. Nursing staff are the guardians for maintaining environmental safety and undertake searches of young people returning to the unit and regular environmental searches to ensure young people have no access to implements used for self-harming. Responding to duress alarms and the emergency administration of parenteral medication is also a common occurrence. Various ways of coordinating care have been trialled. In an effort to increase the likelihood patients will interact with a familiar nurse, the Walker Unit presently organises the nursing workforce into three teams that are allocated specific patients.

Keywords Psychiatric nursing • Adolescent • Inpatients • Risk management

S. Hoare (✉) • S. Ho
Walker Unit, Concord Centre for Mental Health, Concord, NSW, Australia
e-mail: Steve.Hoare@health.nsw.gov.au; Stephen.Ho@health.nsw.gov.au

© The Author(s) 2022
P. Hazell (ed.), *Longer-Term Psychiatric Inpatient Care for Adolescents*, https://doi.org/10.1007/978-981-19-1950-3_6

The Nursing Team

The nursing team at the Walker Unit is an ever changing body of people, with quarterly rotation in junior nurses undertaking their Transition into Mental Health Nursing development year and a generally stable group of CAMHS experienced nurses ranging from three to eight or more years. Approximately half of the regular staff have undertaken some level of post graduate training in child and adolescent mental health.

Leading the nursing team is a Nurse Unit Manager (NUM) and a Clinical Nurse Consultant (CNC), who perform two distinct functions; NUM responsibilities include management of human resources and facilities, staff performance and organisational capacity issues, while the CNC is responsible for clinical issues related to care planning, risk management of patients, organising the referral process and undertaking pre-admission assessments and supporting the milieu of the unit.

The number of staff each shift is based upon the number of patients on the unit, organised as part of the wider hospital on a shift by shift basis, so can range between two and five staff. The night shift is always staffed by two nurses, between Sunday and Thursday one staff member on the afternoon shift starts later to cover a twilight shift to support night staff settle the unit. Because some young people are granted home leave on the weekend, nursing numbers will typically be lower than during the working week. Nursing numbers can be increased to respond to the level of clinical dependency, such as requiring care level one observations to support safety of a young person. There are times when nurses from adult mental health wards are deployed to the Walker Unit to fill staffing shortages.

Supporting Young People

At the Walker Unit, there are three nursing teams of five. Each team is led by an experienced CAMHS Registered Nurse (RN8) or Clinical Nurse Specialist (CNS1). A team is responsible for two to four young people, and the staff in that team become their young person's "Primary Nurses". The rationale for team nursing is to foster, as far is possible, continuity of nursing care and maximise the number of shifts as possible for a young person being nursed by someone familiar with their care. Primary nurses should focus some of their time to develop effective therapeutic relationships with their primary young people; getting to know their interests, likes, dislikes and aspirations for the future. As a relationship is established, nurses can then engage a young person with collaborating in care planning and explore challenges they experience, and evaluate the effectiveness of care plan interventions attempted. Primary nurses typically attend family meetings as a support to the young person, advocate their perspective or provide feedback to family members. Within their primary nurse team there is a "Lead Primary Nurse" for each individual, this role is purposely an administrative one to ensure that care plans, required documentation and reports are kept up-to-date and are accessible.

DAY-TO-DAY ALLOCATION OF NURSING TASKS

The allocation of staff to young people usually also considers the therapeutic relationships between staff and a young person, a young person's level of clinical dependency, previous clinical incidents such as self-harm or verbally hostile or aggressive behaviour as well as the level of experience a staff member has in supporting young people with complex behaviours. Other considerations include staff fatigue, shift patterns worked and recent previous allocation to patients, so there is sharing of the clinical workload. It is not uncommon for young people to express dissatisfaction when they are allocated staff who they are not familiar with, or that they have had challenging experiences with, and therefore being able to explain allocation decisions, both clearly and with diplomacy is a skill required by the nurse in charge. When a young person requires supervision on care level one, within eye-sight or arms reach, additional staff are requested to support this intervention. The supervision is shared amongst all the staff on shift with a maximum two hour period on 1:1 observations. To support the allocations of patient care and other jobs on a shift by shift basis, the nurse in charge works from a diary that has reminders for role and activities required each day, they transcribe their allocations onto a white board in the nursing office visible for all staff to view and know their jobs for the shift.

MANAGING SAFETY ON THE UNIT

Nursing staff are the guardians of the environment and undertake shift by shift safety checks. There are typically several patients on the unit who will scan the environment for opportunities and means to self-harm. As such, nurses must ensure the removal of used linen (ligature risk), cutlery and crockery removal after meals and snacks (cutting risk), ensuring musical instruments and videogames consoles are securely stored when not in use (strings and power cords provide a ligature risk). Young people being admitted or returning from periods of leave must participate in a search before entering the main unit environment to prevent contraband items being brought into the environment. The main focus is implements for self-harm, such as blades or shards of glass, but illicit substances are also "on the radar". There are two levels of search used: PAT and GOWN search. A PAT search involves a declaration if they have contraband items, emptying pockets and bags to nursing staff and handing in any devices or restricted items to be held securely. A GOWN search is a more invasive process and is summarized in Box 6.1.

The decision to use PAT or GOWN search is based on the patient's recent risk history.

Care Planning

The primary nurse team has responsibility to engage the young person in thinking about their care plan and treatment, they have knowledge of the aims of an admission, the strengths and difficulties questionnaire and consumer wellness plans that are completed by young people to guide their understanding of what the content of care plans should be. The Walker Unit has two kinds of care plan; a multidisciplinary (MDT) care plan and specific or targeted care plan. It is the second that is usually created between nursing staff and the young people. Specific or targeted care plans

---

Box 6.1 Elements of a GOWN Search

- Two staff undertake the search—of the young person's preferred gender
- Staff gain consent
- Conduct in a bathroom
- Ask young person to hand in any contraband items
- Young person disrobes to underwear and puts on hospital gown
- Young person removes underwear
- Clothing searched by staff
- Visual person search and metal detector search conducted
- Young person dresses

typically aim to increase a young person's skills in managing a task or situation more independently through practice or attempting different strategies. The structure of the care plan used is depicted in Fig. 6.1.

The first page includes identification of young person; name, Medical Record Number (MRN), care plan number and a care plan title. The title of the care plan should be relatable to the young person and be written using language easily understood. An example would be "Building tolerance to my emotions and distress" rather than "Managing aggressive behaviour". The title of a care plan is often the beginning of the "sales pitch" used by staff to persuade a young person to work in collaboration with their team. The young person or family's observation is next and details in their own words what they see as the challenge in their situation that requires support. The team adds their observations of the same. A rationale for the care plan is given in "Identified need" section, which guides the young person as to what benefits may be achieved by working through the care plan with the team. Lastly, the "Goal" of the care plan should be linked to the overall aims of the admission. These two sections are written in "recovery focused" language, offering hope and optimism that changes can be made. Coffey et al. (Coffey et al., 2019) support the recovery focus in care planning and choice of language to support consumers.

The second page of the Care Plan (see Fig. 6.2) lists interventions that should be used to work through the presenting situation. These interventions are written in sequence and guide staff what should be done and how. Interventions take into account the wishes of a young person.

If a young person's behaviour raises safety concerns, decisions for interventions can be taken by nursing staff. Actions can include relocating the young person to a more contained area of the unit, increasing the level of direct observations, activating the duress system to increase staff availability, and administering PRN medication. On occasion, this may require the use of restraint. Restrictive practices are only deployed to maintain safety if less intrusive interventions have been ineffective.

Care plans are developed consistent with the principles of trauma informed care, offering choice to a young person, empowerment through self-determination, collaboration throughout the experience, developing trustworthiness and maintaining safety, both physically and psychologically. The nursing staff have a care planning resource folder that includes

Walker Unit - CCMH
CARE PLAN

Name: Angela Raynor	MRN: 1234567
Unit: Walker	Care Plan No: 2
Care Plan Title: Night time routine and good sleep hygiene.	

Young Person / Family Observations:

Angela reports experiencing increased anxiety and racing thoughts at night. Angela often has nightmares and avoids sleeping. After a nightmare Angela ruminates about hurting herself.

Angela likes to use sensory distraction at bedtime to help settle her to sleep. She also likes her room to be sprayed with Lavender spray.

Team Observations:

Angela struggles to have a consistent sleeping pattern and experiences heightened anxiety at night. She has a changeable sleep pattern, and there have been nights when she has not managed to sleep despite having medications, and she becomes distressed during the night. Angela struggles to manage her distress and at during these times can act upon her urges to hurt herself; head-banging or attempting to self-strangulate/use ligatures.

Identified Need:
To develop a regular sleeping pattern which supports Angela to feel safe and have a restful night sleep.
To prepare her body for getting to sleep and manage any anxiety she experiences.
To reduce the reliance on medications to aid sleep.

Goal(s):

To achieve a functioning restorative sleeping pattern that supports Angela to effectively manage her emotions and activities to her best capacity.

Review Due Date:	Reviewed By:	Review Due Date:	Reviewed By:
22/3/25	A.M		
29/3/25	C. NURSE		

Fig. 6.1 Example of a care plan (p. 1)

Walker Unit - CCMH
CARE PLAN

| Name: Angela Raynor | MRN: 1234567 |
| | Care Plan No: 2 |

Interventions:

Angela and staff to follow the night time routine as outlined below:

Angela remains on care level 3 throughout the night.
1. Angela to have supper between 19:30-20:00hrs (cereal/toast or popped corn and milk drink).
2. Angela to have nocte medications between 20:00-20:30hrs.
   a. Mirtazapine
   b. 20mg Promethazine PRN
3. Angela to shower and change into bed clothes between 20:00-21:00hrs. Towels and day clothes to be stored in locked cupboard.
4. Staff should spray scented spray in her bedroom (Kept in office).
5. Angela to retire to her bedroom between 21:00-21:30hrs and undertake a relaxing activity:
   a. Reading on kindle (Phone).
   b. Listening to music/soothing sounds.
   c. Diary/journaling.
   Angela can undertake the activity until 22:30hrs when she must try and sleep.
6. If Angela is not asleep by 23:00hrs, she can be offered 25mg Quetiapine PRN.
7. Angela should attempt to sleep following medication administration, mobile devices should be collected at 23:00hrs. IPad can be left with soothing sounds whilst trying to settle to sleep.
8. If Angela is still awake after 45 minutes, staff can offer her 1mg Lorazepam PRN.
9. The use of PRN Promethazine should be reviewed and consider reduction once an established pattern of sleep has been achieved.
10. If Angela becomes distressed at night, staff should support her following care plan 1; building tolerance to my emotions care plan.
11. Staff will review this care plan with Angela fortnightly.

Staff Name: G. Nurse	Staff Signature:
Qualifications: RN	Date: 15/03/2025
Young Person Signature: Monica Raynn	Parents Signature:

Fig. 6.2 Example of a care plan (p. 2)

Table 6.1   List of care plan templates

No	Care Plan Title	Comments
1	Building tolerance to emotional distress and staying safe	For supporting young people who self-harm, includes de-escalation tree
2	Help when I'm losing my cool	For supporting young people with known patterns of escalating behaviour, early warning signs to unsafe behaviours
3	"Help me" when I'm angry	To guide staff in managing aggressive behaviour, towards environment, self or others
4	Physical health needs as important as mental health	For supporting young people with physical health problems and are at risk of metabolic syndrome
5	Supporting healthy dietary intake and healthy lifestyle choices	To guide young people who have disordered eating behaviours or are on a weight management plan
6	Night time routine and good sleep hygiene	To develop effective sleep hygiene and night routines
7	Monitoring mental state and medication efficacy	To support young people starting new antipsychotic/antidepressant/mood stabilizing medications
8	Supporting Young Person (YP) experiencing positive symptoms of psychosis	To guide young people and staff to manage positive symptoms of illness effectively, and support engagement in program or create individual program
9	Supporting safe home leave and return to unit	Detailing strategies for families to manage safety at home, telephone or additional support and level of search on return to the Walker unit
10	School integration care plan	Including contact details for support, helpful activities, strategies in school, supervision needs and transport details

ten template care plans, providing them with guides as to what should be included in care plans for specific situations, so that they can discuss and individualise care plans with a young person. The template titles are listed in Table 6.1.

MOTIVATING YOUNG PEOPLE TO ENGAGE IN CARE PLANS

The Walker Unit runs a continuous achievement level system consisting of five different achievement levels; bronze; silver; gold; platinum and diamond. Each level has different privileges and restrictions; lower levels having increased restrictions and less privileges and higher levels less

LEVEL	Mobile Phone and Electronics	1:1 Outings	SIM card	Negotiated Bedtime	Group Outings	Unescorted leave to Toms, Thurs markets & Riverside	Kitchen	Unescorted Leave	Room Privileges	Sleep-ins
Diamond	✓	✓	✓	✓	✓	✓	✓	✓	✓	✓
Platinum	✓	✓	✓	✓	✓	✓	✓	✓		
Gold	✓	✓	✓	✓	✓					
Silver	✓	✓								
Bronze										

Fig. 6.3 Summary of level system

restrictions and more privileges (See Fig. 6.3). Privileges include access to mobile devices, SIM cards, attending outings, going on daily walks, kitchen access and unescorted leave off the unit. If a young person displays unsafe behaviour such as aggression towards others, damage to property or deliberate self-harm requiring medical intervention a young person is placed on bronze level for 24 hours, this has the most restricted access to privileges, if they manage the 24 hour period without repeat of the behaviours they move back to silver level.

This achievement level system was initially designed with the young people and acts as a positive reinforcement for the young people. A young person's level reflects their effort in engaging in the treatment program, following their care plans and managing their safety. Movement up and down the levels provides the team, but particularly the nursing staff with a tool to reward effort, but also to provide natural consequences for behaviours displayed. There are occasions where a young person's capacity to follow the level system requires adjustments; so, a care plan is created to specify these circumstances and adjustments.

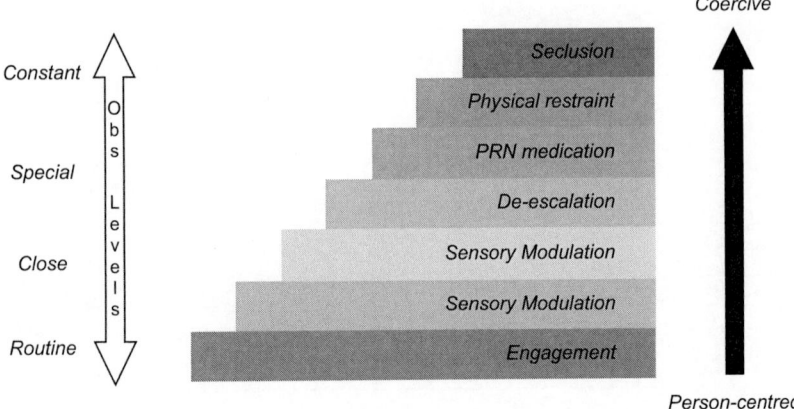

Fig. 6.4 Hierarchy of nursing intervention. (Reproduced with permission from Spencer, S. (2017). *Nursing Responses and Interventions for Episodes of Adolescent Distress in an Acute Child and Adolescent Mental Health Inpatient Unit: An Interpretive Descriptive Study.* (Unpublished Doctoral Dissertation) University of Newcastle)

OBSERVATIONS FOR SAFETY AND BEING PRESENT

Physical presence on the floor requires that effective allocation of duties and sufficient staffing is maintained. Being present and engaging with young people is emotionally labour intensive (Forster & Smedley, 2019a; Forster & Smedley, 2019b) and requires staff to be interested in the young people, and be able to engage in age appropriate dialogue, or participate in light hearted fun situations such as playing games or activities. Senior nursing staff use Spence's (Spencer, 2017) model of nursing interventions to promote active engagement and demonstrate interventions becoming more coercive or restrictive when reflecting on practice (see Fig. 6.4).

At the same time as offering diversional activities, staff should be vigilant to observe for changes in behaviours of young people and be ready to intervene when a young person is "triggered" by something or someone. Young people at the Walker Unit have limited choice as to where they spend time and whom is in their vicinity, therefore negative interactions can and do occur between them. Staff need to be able to carefully manage interactions between young people, provide activities that can be inclusive such as board games, movies or card games and invite the whole group of young people to participate. For many young people simply being invited to be involved can help change their feeling within the environment. Having an allocated staff member to monitor the whereabouts of young people each hour shares the responsibility of locating all young people. Closing down the environment dependent on the ward activities is another way of simplifying this task and ensure everyone is visually accounted for, an example is at night time, the wider unit is closed and locked to bring activities for young people into the main lounge, bedroom and bathroom corridors and focus on completing the night time routines.

Clinical Supervision for Nursing Staff

There are a number of ways clinical supervision is offered at the Walker Unit for nursing staff; monthly group clinical supervision for nursing staff only, fortnightly whole team systemic clinical supervision, monthly incident review meetings, hot and cold debriefs following an incident and individual clinical supervision. Nursing group supervision is undertaken by an external supervisor and is independent of the NUM and the CNC. The nature of the young people's presentations, managing the therapeutic milieu, engaging with the young people, the application of the level system, sitting with young people in distress, or de-escalating situational behaviours all have an impact on staffs emotional availability. Decisions made amongst team members can often spur different personal views and perspectives on treatment which ignite passionate and sometimes emotional responses between staff, clinical supervision on all levels is one way to discuss and explore these situations, identify and articulate nursing interventions and any resolutions needed (Forster & Smedley, 2019b).

References

Coffey, M., Hannigan, B., Barlow, S., Cartwright, M., Cohen, R., Faulkner, A., Jones, A., & Simpson, A. (2019). Recovery-focused mental health care planning and co-ordination in acute inpatient mental health settings: A cross national comparative mixed methods study. *BMC Psychiatry, 19*(1), 115. https://doi.org/10.1186/s12888-019-2094-7

Forster, C., & Smedley, K. (2019a). Understanding the nature of mental health nursing within CAMHS PICU:1. Identifying nursing interventions that contribute to the recovery journey of young people. *Journal of Psychiatric Intensive Care, 15*(2), 87–102. https://doi.org/10.20299/jpi.2019.012

Forster, C., & Smedley, K. (2019b). Understanding the nature of mental health nursing within CAMHS PICU: 2. Staff experience and support needs. *Journal of Psychiatric Intensive Care, 15*(2), 103–115. https://doi.org/10.20299/jpi.2019.013

Spencer, S. (2017). *Nursing responses and interventions for episodes of adolescent distress in an acute child and adolescent mental health inpatient unit: An interpretive descriptive study.* University of Newcastle.

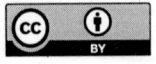

CHAPTER 7

Learning Centre and School Reintegration

Isabelle Feijo, Steve Hoare, Amanda Scali,
and Jennifer Shumack

Abstract The Learning Centre is an important part of the Walker Unit Program as it provides structure to the day and helps the young person to regain confidence in their cognitive ability after often a long absence in education and learning, and it supports the young person in the transition to an appropriate educational setting after discharge.

Keywords Adolescent • Inpatients • Education • Distance • Patient discharge

I. Feijo (✉) • S. Hoare
Walker Unit, Concord Centre for Mental Health, Concord, NSW, Australia
e-mail: Isabelle.Feijo@health.nsw.gov.au; Steve.Hoare@health.nsw.gov.au

A. Scali • J. Shumack
Rivendell School, Concord, NSW, Australia
e-mail: Amanda.Robinson14@det.nsw.gov.au; Jennifer.Shumack@det.nsw.gov.au

© The Author(s) 2022
P. Hazell (ed.), *Longer-Term Psychiatric Inpatient Care for Adolescents*, https://doi.org/10.1007/978-981-19-1950-3_7

INTRODUCTION

The model of delivery of the Walker Unit Learning Centre is the result of an evolution of a collaboration between NSW Health and the NSW Department of Education. Hospital Schools had been established in NSW since 1976 when a schoolroom, in partnership with the Department of Education was provided in the new Prince of Wales Children's Hospital (Department of Education, 2021). The model of having a classroom within an inpatient unit developed later and started to take shape after it was strongly advocated by health and education experts to ensure that students in inpatient units had access to education in line with Article 28 of the United Nations Convention on the Rights of the Child (UNICEF, 2021).

PRIOR TO ADMISSION

Education is a core component that is considered prior to the young person's admission to the Walker Unit. When the Walker team go out to assess the young person (see Chap. 4), they gather information about the young person's educational history. As most young people have a long and relapsing illness, their educational pathway has been disrupted and it is not unusual that they have been absent from school and learning for months or years. As school is an essential part of their recovery process, the Walker Program supports all students, independent of their capacity and level to regain an educational pathway. The process of transitioning the young person from the hospital-based learning centre to a school in the community is referred to as integration.

FIRST WEEK

On admission, the young person is introduced to the Learning Centre using principles of graded exposure to support anxiety and adjust to the environment and new people. How a young person copes with this transition at the start of admission provides an indication as to how integration into a community educational facility towards discharge should be managed. The patient is assessed to determine their level of educational functioning. The education team, together with the health team decide early in the admission what the optimal discharge educational destination could be. Many young people would have difficulty reintegrating into the mainstream school system and an application or Access Request may be submitted in order to access a placement in a School for Specific Purposes (SSP).

When a young person commences attending the Learning Centre, the Walker education team focuses on engagement, information gathering and academic assessment. There is liaison with the patient's previous educational placements to assist the teachers in developing the young person's academic programme. Previous school history can also be helpful in informing psychiatric diagnosis, and assessment of function.

FORMULATION AND CARE PLANNING

In the third or fourth week of admission, the mini team assigned to work with the patient undertake a Formulation and Care Planning meeting (see Chap. 5). Teachers attend the first of these meetings in order to gather information that is necessary to support the young person in the Learning Centre, and also to feedback to the health team regarding any information gathered around schooling. The discharge pathway is considered, including the educational pathway. Once the school pathway has been determined, the team supports the young person's family in order to achieve a successful outcome regarding schooling. The health team may request the Walker teachers to attend family meetings in order to assist parents with acceptance around educational planning.

LEARNING CENTRE

Within the Walker Unit, there are two classrooms called Learning Centres. All students are required to attend school to the best of their capacity every morning from Monday to Friday. The Learning Centre schedule comprises two 1.5 hour periods each week day during term time and is part of the therapeutic treatment programme. During school holidays, the same periods in the day are filled with diversionary activities facilitated by educationally trained staff. Whilst young people are attending the Learning Centre, there is always a member of nursing staff present to observe and support the young people to focus on and attempt school tasks. Some young people can avoid schooling tasks through a variety of challenging behaviours. Nursing staff are there to support young people who may escalate in their behaviour, move them out of the environment, de-escalate and resolve before re-engaging in learning.

The Walker education team is staffed by two teachers and two school learning support officers (SLSOs) with support provided by the principal and school counsellor from the adjacent Rivendell School. The Walker education team are also closely involved in the Rivendell School community and engage in whole school activities including professional learning and workshops on a weekly basis.

Teachers

Teachers work with the young person and all stakeholders in order to develop an academic programme, including teaching and learning activities and individual plans to support the young person. Teachers liaise with various stakeholders in support of the young person. They attend weekly Case Review meetings and provide feedback to the multidisciplinary team about student progress in the Learning Centre and during integration. They maintain regular contact with the home school and their future educational setting. Teachers may also attend family meetings to discuss educational matters.

Teachers also manage the processes that involve the continuity of the young person's education, such as ensuring they have evidence to achieve their Record of School Achievement (RoSA) at the end of year 10, and assisting in the application for special provisions for those in year 12 undertaking their exit examinations. Teachers may also assist students with pursuing alternative vocational settings and coordinating the Access Request process between schools when it is decided by the treating team that an alternate school placement is needed.

School Learning Support Officers (SLSOs)

SLSOs fulfil a number of administrative roles including recording attendance, preparing resources and organising the equipment in the Learning Centre to ensure that the environment is well equipped and safe. Another key role of the SLSOs is to support student engagement and achievement in the Learning Centre. They work 1:1 with students to support them in their learning and contribute to all key Learning Centre activities.

School Reintegration

Once a young person's mental illness has stabilised, the treating team will support the young person by facilitating a slow and progressive integration from hospital to school. Once a school has been confirmed for the young person, the Walker teachers arrange an integration meeting that usually occurs at the receiving school. The meeting is attended by the treating team, the Walker teacher and the key contacts at the school. The integration meeting helps inform the school integration plan and care plan. Close communication is maintained between the Walker Unit teachers and the receiving setting throughout the whole integration process until discharge.

School integration plans are staged, starting with shorter time periods and in favoured subject lessons or with support staff available. The aim is to gradually increase their exposure to the environment, to other students and staff and for longer periods in the day. The frequency of integration days gradually increases up to a maximum of three days. Walker teachers gather timely feedback from schools during the integration and communicate this to the health team to ensure all parties are up to date with progress. Typically, the integration process is spread over five weeks.

Ahead of school integration, a care plan is developed jointly by education and health staff that includes strategies for recognising and managing the early warning signs that the young person is struggling. The care plan will have self-help strategies for the young person, and guidance for staff on what to do if the situation escalates. Interventions may include sensory modulation activities, time out periods, meeting a mentor or staff member, contact with the Walker Unit or parents and use of PRN (pro re nata or "as needed") medication. Contact details of key support people are highlighted in the care plan Figs. 7.1 and 7.2.

Transport to and from integration is ideally undertaken by parents or carers of the young person, but if the school is within reasonable proximity to the Walker Unit nursing staff may support the initial stages of integration. An ongoing need for a clinician to support the integration is an indicator that the young person is not yet ready for discharge.

Walker Unit - CCMH
CARE PLAN

Name: Angela Raynor	MRN: 1234567
Unit: Walker	Issue No: 8
Problem Title: Successful school integration care plan.	

Young Person / Family Observations:

Angela is anxious about being in a new school environment, with unfamiliar staff and students. She worries about being able to explain to others where she has been during her hospital admission, and that she may find the work too hard.

Team Observations:

Angela has been working in the learning centre at Walker with minimal support or supervision required from education staff. Angela works best when having a task set for 30 minutes and having a break for 10 minutes to listen to music and prepare for the next task. When Angela is finding the work difficult she finds it hard to ask for help, but has used a visual prompt, placing her pencil case upside down on the table to signal to staff she needs assistance.

Identified Need:

Maintain Angela's focus on tasks set in the classroom.
Support her interactions in meeting other students.
Respond to anxiety with helpful distraction activities.

Goal(s):

Support Angela to engage in education activities at her new school.
To help Angela to get to know her new teachers and work with them to complete tasks.
To get to know new students in her classroom and develop supportive relationships.

Review Due Date:	Reviewed By:	Review Due Date:	Reviewed By:
22	3	25	G N URSE		

Fig. 7.1   Example of a school integration care plan (p. 1)

Walker Unit - CCMH
CARE PLAN

Name: Angela Raynor	MRN: 1234567
	Issue No: 8

Interventions:

Angela has a 5 week integration plan to progressively increase her attendance at her new school. This will initially be supported by nursing staff for the first 3 sessions, then her mother will take over supporting her to school.

Handing over care process:
Nursing staff/then mom to take Angela to school reception and meet her school counsellor and talk through the plan for her day. Her school counsellor will take her to classes.

Early Warning Signs for distress:
- Angela can stare at her lap top and stop communicating with others.
- Angela becomes fidgety when she is in class and struggling with her thoughts or feelings.
- She can begin to pace around the room.
- Angela will place her pencil case upside down on her desk if she requires help.

Helpful distraction activities/sensory modulation activities:
- Angela finds using a fidget spinner helpful to support her to complete her school work.
- She finds listening to music through her headphones supportive.
- If she has finished a task, having some time outside to shoot basketball hoops for 10 minutes is useful.

Time out agreements in school:
30 minutes on task followed by a 10 minute break outside is helpful before starting the next task.

Supervision needs (Health/education staff / bathroom use):
Angela can use the bathroom during her breaks between completing tasks. She does not require bathroom supervision by staff.

Escalation for support:
Education staff – School counsellor Liz (0412345678) or Assistant Principle Jenny (0423456789)
Health staff – Walker staff (9787 4561)
Family – Mother (Doreen) 0456789101.

Staff Name: G. Nurse	Staff Signature:
Qualifications: RN	Date: 15/3/25
Young Person Signature:	Parents Signature:

Fig. 7.2 Example of a school integration care plan (p. 2)

Discharge

In preparation for discharge from hospital, the Walker education team communicate the details of a young person's mental health treating team in the community to the school to assist with continuity of care. Sometimes it will be agreed with a school that the young person will continue a negotiated partial attendance plan beyond discharge, or they may return to school full time. Prior to discharge, a farewell is organised for the young person by the Walker team. As a part of the farewell, Walker education staff present the young person with their academic report, a scroll that is co-written by the education staff and the young person's peers and any other certificates they have earned during their time at the Walker Unit.

References

Department of Education. (2021). *Recollections of Prince of Wales hospital school and the Sydney Children's Hospital School.* Retrieved 11 October, 2021, from https://sydchnhos-s.schools.nsw.gov.au/about-our-school/our-history.html

UNICEF. (2021). *United Nations convention on the rights of the child.* Retrieved 11 October, 2021, from https://www.unicef.org.au/upload/unicef/media/unicef-simplified-convention-child-rights.pdf

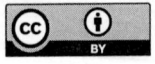

CHAPTER 8

Family Therapy

Karen Sarmiento and Isabelle Feijo

Abstract The hospitalisation of a young person, particularly over an extended period of time, inevitably impacts on the entire family. Prior to admission to the Walker Unit, the young person and their family will have typically engaged with several other inpatient services and will have been exposed to a range of psychological and pharmacological treatments, with mixed results. However when discharged into the same unchanged family milieu, a deterioration can occur resulting in rehospitalisation and the need for further intensive care. By the time families arrive at a Walker admission, they are probably suffering treatment fatigue due to the impact of long hospitalisation and the impact of chronic mental illness. This needs to be overcome.

Keywords Adolescent • Inpatients • Family therapy • Parent-child relations • Siblings

K. Sarmiento • I. Feijo (✉)
Walker Unit, Concord Centre for Mental Health, Concord, NSW, Australia
e-mail: Karen.Sarmiento@health.nsw.gov.au; Isabelle.Feijo@health.nsw.gov.au

© The Author(s) 2022
P. Hazell (ed.), *Longer-Term Psychiatric Inpatient Care for Adolescents*, https://doi.org/10.1007/978-981-19-1950-3_8

Introduction

"Both clinical experience and research tell us that the therapeutic alliance between staff, children and their parents needs to be positive if the child is to have a good chance of making progress during the course of their admission"(Gross & Goldin, 2008). Family therapy plays an integral part in the recovery process and has a beneficial impact on the lives of adolescents and their families by improving functioning and quality of life (Merritts, 2017). For these reasons, family therapy is an essential part of the Walker Unit treatment programme delivered in conjunction with other treatment modalities. Our aim is to support the young person and their entire family system to change, so that a therapeutic discharge into a modified (improved) home environment can occur. Groundwork for family therapy is laid during the admission process described in Chap. 4. It begins with the assessment meeting at the mental health facility (if they are an inpatient) or at the local community mental health centre. To emphasise the importance of engagement by all family members, we require, from the outset, the participation of all family members living in the same household.

Family Therapy

The Walker Unit family therapy frame consists of weekly sessions. Sometimes the treating team will meet with a subset of the family (for example only the siblings) for specific therapeutic goals. For families who live a great distance from the unit we offer a hybrid of face-to-face and virtual meetings. Virtual meetings have also been used extensively during the COVID pandemic (see Chap. 20). We offer divorced or separated parents the option of being seen separately. For therapeutic reasons they may, however, be required to attend sessions together on some occasions.

A co-therapy approach is taken with sessions led by the consultant psychiatrist and a psychologist or social worker. The psychiatrist in training assigned to the patient is also a member of the family therapy team. Sessions may also be attended by the patient's primary nurse, and by students on clinical placement. Therapy can follow several different approaches, such as structural, systemic and multigenerational with consideration given to the underlying capacity demonstrated by the family to engage in the therapeutic process.

The main task of the first session is to construct a genogram which includes information about the quality of the relationship between members, personality traits/ characteristics, hobbies and interests, employment status, legal issues and education. Special attention is given to parental upbringing, past domestic violence, serious family illness, migration, traumatic events such as deaths, suicide and abuse as well as physical and mental health history. The process enables us to identify patterns of behaviour and relationships across generations. Figure 8.1 provides an example of how a genogram is recorded.

Constructing the genogram may take one or a several sessions and remains a resource we refer back to throughout treatment. We build on the genogram work by obtaining a developmental history of the patient. Obtaining a clearer understanding of early childhood experiences and how the young person and family managed transitions from preschool to primary school to high school, provides insight into the evolution of the patient's difficulties and how the family system has responded. As part of this exploratory process, family members are invited to share their thoughts and opinions on what they would like to see change or be different. A key aspect of this exercise is the building of an effective therapeutic alliance (Goplolan et al., 2010) which is necessary to hold and contain the family during difficult stages of the work, particularly when the young person is experiencing a set-back in their recovery. The family's level of engagement

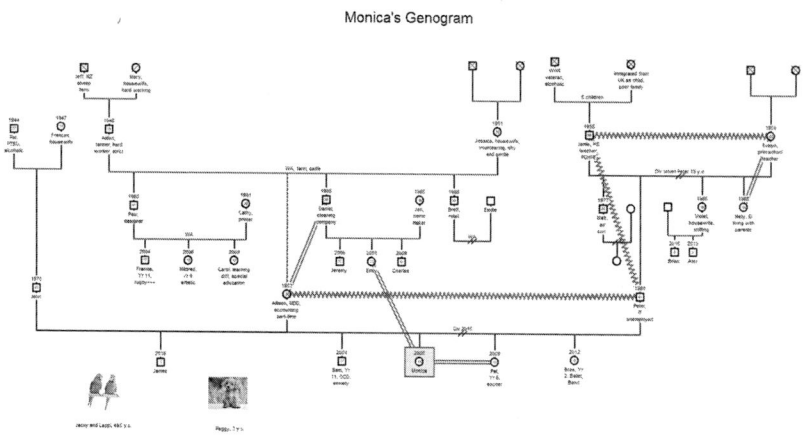

Fig. 8.1 Example of a genogram

and participation in the genogram exploration helps guide our treatment approach, as those who demonstrate openness, spontaneity and some reflective capacity are the most suitable for systemic work.

Ongoing sessions consist of both therapeutic exploration as well as the discussion of more practical matters such as medication changes, voluntary/involuntary admission status and weekend leave arrangements. However the main focus remains on the systemic process such as ongoing work on improving communication within the family, helping the family to problem solve difficulties arising during leave (self-harm, suicide attempts, absconding), and helping the parents to work collaboratively, re-instating the hierarchy (de-parentification of the identified patient). After one month of admission, the family is provided with a preliminary treatment plan that offers detailed information on the presenting issues, goals of treatment and estimated discharge date (see Chap. 5 for more detail). Care is taken to go through the plan with the patient and their family in a collaborative manner. All members are encouraged to give honest feedback with specific consideration given to anything that needs to be added or changed. In further sessions, we work with the family on systemic and relational goals that have been observed to contribute to the evolution of the young person's difficulties or that play a part in perpetuating unhelpful dynamics.

A home visit is conducted at least once during the period of admission. The aim is to meet the family in their own environment to get a better sense of what it is like for the young person to be at home; it affords an opportunity to learn things that are not readily accessible by meeting the family on the unit. It can provide a rich source of information surrounding the level of emotional and physical care available which is often observed through how warm and welcoming the environment is. This includes levels of basic cleanliness, how light or dark the place is, whether there is sufficient and appropriate furniture and so on. It also gives information on the neighbourhood, proximity to community resources and the school, whether the household is permeable (drop in visits from neighbours, relatives) or impermeable (seemingly isolated). Moreover, we get to see and interact with the pets, we see artworks produced by the children stuck on the fridge door and other personal effects such as family photos that tell stories we wouldn't otherwise know. Even the car journey with the young person can be very informative as we get to listen to their music and discuss matters that would not be discussed at the Unit. Home visits also allow for the therapy team to acknowledge the weekly effort made by families and provides an opportunity for us to meet with other members who have been unable to attend sessions in the hospital. This may be due to anxiety and avoidance, physical/mental illness or other practical matters such as work.

Leave is introduced in a gradual manner (see Fig. 8.2); owing to safety concerns, a young person's home and community leave may have to be reduced or ceased. A central task of the Walker family therapy process includes the reintroduction of leave in a gradual and safe way. The home visit sets the groundwork for this process. In situations where there is high anxiety regarding leave at home, a visit can provide a necessary first step of exposure. Usually, the psychiatrist, family therapist, registrar and nurse attend the home with the young person and act as a containment team to buffer interactions with the family, and assist with any risk issues that might emerge for example, the young person absconding or engaging in self-harm. An important part of the family therapy at this stage includes assisting the family and young person to problem-solve difficulties that emerge, exploring how reactive responses may be contributing to the escalation of conflict and supporting members to tolerate challenging behaviours and difficult feelings aroused as a part of the leave. A family chain

Leave Journey at Walker

Increasing ability to self-regulate and participation in the ward's activities

	Stage 1 Settling in	Stage 2 Ground leave	Stage 3 Day leave	Stage 4 Weekend leave	Stage 5 Weekday leave	
Situation	• 7 days stay-in • Visitors welcome	• Up to 2 hours leave • Within the grounds of the hospital (Rivendell and Concord Hospital)	• Up to 1 hours leave (gradual increase) • Can be leave to home or local places • Close supervision recommended during leave to **home** or local places	• Up to 3 nights (Fri-Mon) • Home/relative home • Motel/hotel (for families form rural area)	• Another overnight leave during the week on top of weekend leave	**Stage 6 – Discharge Planning**
Suggestions	• Courtyard picnic • Board games • Table tennis • Watching a movie • Meals together	• Walks • Picnic • Ball games	Activities to do at home: Watching a movie, sharing a meal, cooking/baking, playing games, walks Local leave: ➢ Rhodes Waterfront ➢ Majors Bay Rd Café ➢ Kokoda Track ➢ Bicentennial park ➢ Aquatic centre	• Discuss and plan weekend schedule/ activities with the team	• School integration from home • Independent travelling	

Low stimulus activities →→→ *Increasing stimulation*

Fig. 8.2 Stages of leave

analysis may be conducted to better understand interactional sequences contributing to dysfunctional dynamics, thereby bringing awareness to unconscious patterns of behaviour and overall areas of being stuck. At times, it becomes necessary to support members to adjust their expectations regarding the amount of change that is possible within the scope of the admission, for example accepting a reduction in the level of serious self-harm rather than self-harm ceasing altogether.

In sessions, a variety of techniques can be used to gather information and to encourage members to reflect on their experiences such as role play, use of a white board, using figurines and drawings. Every effort is made to amplify family strengths and the positive changes that members are making, no matter how small. Tracking these changes across the admission can be helpful in assisting members to recognise their achievements and to observe the skill building that has developed over time. In the case of a young person being under the care of the Minister and living in an Out of Home Care arrangement, the family therapy team works closely with the carers and child protection case managers to support them in the safe transition back into their care.

School Integration (See Also Chap. 7)

Once the young person's mental state has stabilised we begin exploring appropriate educational options for the young person. This can often involve applying to a school for specific purposes (SSP) for specialised emotional and educational support. When a suitable pathway has been identified the Walker teacher and treating team meet with the school (if possible in person) to discuss the young person's needs and put together an integration plan. The family and young person also attend this meeting and equally contribute to the plan that is put in place. Much like home leave, attending an outside school is considered leave within the community and an integral part of the overall treatment programme.

Discharge and Handover

Throughout the young person's admission, the treatment plan is periodically reviewed by the family and team to monitor progress and make necessary adjustments. This treatment plan includes the estimated discharge date and the decision if this should remain the same or change, depending on the young person's progress and level of engagement in the programme. As discharge draws nearer it becomes vital that we prepare the family for this reality, and ensure that there is sufficient time within the therapy to effectively discuss concerns, and examine any remaining work that needs to be done.

REFERENCES

Goplolan, G., Goldstein, L., Klingenstein, K., Sicher, C., Blake, C., & McKay, M. M. (2010). Engaging families into child mental health treatment: Updates and special considerations. *Journal of the Canadian Academy of Child and Adolescent Psychiatry, 19*(3), 182–196.

Gross, V., & Goldin, J. (2008). Dynamics and dilemmas in working with families in inpatient CAMH services. *Clinical Child Psychology and Psychiatry, 13*(3), 449–461.

Merritts, A. N. (2017). Emerging family therapy models utilized in residential settings. In J. D. Christenson & A. N. Merritts (Eds.), *Family therapy with adolescents in residential treatment. Intervention and research.* Springer.

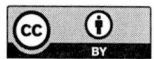

CHAPTER 9

Group Therapies

Fran Nielsen, Polly Kwan, and Nina Mather

Abstract The group therapy programme at the Walker Unit uses a multi-modal approach including verbal, non-verbal, and physical elements. The programme draws on expertise from a range of professional disciplines. The group programme provides therapeutic clinical intervention rather than activity or distraction-based programmes, providing structure and containment as well as cultivating engagement in the therapeutic process and therapy skill building, navigating interpersonal dynamics. Being in a contained unit, the spaces on the ward are also used to facilitate a therapeutic environment during groups. Toward the end of the admissions adolescents and their families may adopt a similarly structured programme or routine including skills and strategies, to assist with their transition from hospital and maintain therapeutic gains achieved from their admission.

Keywords Adolescent • Inpatients • Psychotherapy, Group •
Peer group

F. Nielsen (✉) • P. Kwan • N. Mather
Walker Unit, Concord Centre for Mental Health, Concord, NSW, Australia
e-mail: Fran.Nielsen@health.nsw.gov.au; Polly.Kwan@health.nsw.gov.au;
Nina.Mather@health.nsw.gov.au

© The Author(s) 2022
P. Hazell (ed.), *Longer-Term Psychiatric Inpatient Care for
Adolescents*, https://doi.org/10.1007/978-981-19-1950-3_9

INTRODUCTION

There is a general understanding that children and adolescents develop their self-awareness by making contact with others, equally the sharing of social and cultural knowledge is valuable for personal development (Bo et al., 2017; Rippa, 2016). As in the community, it is common within adolescent mental health units for young people to spend much of their time in one group interaction or another, in school as well as in formal and informal group activities (Griffith, 2010). At the Walker Unit, we acknowledge the importance of group learning, especially with difficult to engage youth who have been isolated from their peers and the community for extended periods. Given many of the young people admitted to the unit have experienced adversity it has been crucial to apply principles of trauma informed care in their treatment (Gudiño et al., 2014).

GROUP THERAPY IN THE WALKER PROGRAMME

Young people admitted to the Walker Unit commonly display emotional and behavioral dysregulation which undermines their capacity to function socially. Other interpersonal difficulties include avoidance, ambivalence, and ambiguity within relationships. Most will have a prior history of unstable relationships in their peer groups and families. Our group therapy programme has been designed to target these difficulties and build the young person's capacity to engage. While the overall structure of group therapy is maintained, there is day to day flexibility to respond to the specific needs of the current patient cohort.

Young people with complex trauma and mental health presentations commonly have difficulties "verbalising" their distress or emotions safely (Chapman, 2014; Cozolino, 2002; Van der Kolk, 2015). The Walker Unit uses a mix of "verbal" and "non-verbal" interventions in the group therapy program. For example, young people are encouraged to take "action" (e.g. body movements, sensory interactions, art and music making) to engage, participate and communicate during the therapy groups. We aim to deliver one verbal and one non-verbal group a day so the young people can engage in therapy through a variety of ways.

A MULTIDISCIPLINARY AND INTERDISCIPLINARY APPROACH

The aims of the therapy groups are to promote social engagement, health literacy, and skills building such as, distress tolerance, emotional regulation, communication, and self-care. Part of the role of the group facilitators is to manage the group dynamics, support the emotions of the young person and expand their window of tolerance. More importantly, the group provides a space for the young people to belong and support their basic needs for interpersonal contact with their peers (Garrick & Ewashen, 2001). In order to promote a greater sense of security and privacy and maintain consistency, some of the groups are closed to observers such as other staff or students (e.g. art psychotherapy group, what's the feeling group, and teenage life group).

Some of the most established groups as outlined in Fig. 9.1:

1. The 'What's the Feeling' group is conducted by the senior social worker and clinical nurse specialist. It supports patients to reflect on their internal world (feelings and emotions), and facilitates the process of using words to describe their experience and to sit with the corresponding discomfort. Scenarios are used as a tool to initiate discussion and to provide opportunities for the consideration of alternate ways of viewing and responding to situations/feeling states.

2. The 'Sports group' is facilitated by experienced nursing staff, and an exercise physiologist when available. This promotes physical and metabolic health, and encourages the young people to nurture a positive body image.

3. The 'Art Psychotherapy Group' facilitates non-verbal self-expression for young people using art materials with the goal to integrate a discussion on thoughts and feelings after the art making. This is supported by a registered senior art therapist (See Chap. 11).

4. The 'Out of Your Comfort Zone' or 'Play Therapy' groups are inter-changeable, depending on the cohort. If the cohort is generally high functioning, the 'Out of Your Comfort Zone' introduces Dialectical Behavior Therapy principles to help develop distress tolerance and awareness. If the cohort is generally low functioning, the 'Play Therapy' group enhances positive relationships between the young people through verbal and non-verbal communication.

Walker Unit - Group Therapy Program

	Monday	Tuesday	Wednesday	Thursday	Friday	Saturday	Sunday
8.30am	Get up and Breakfast	Get up and Breakfast	Get up and Breakfast	Get up and Breakfast	Get up and Breakfast	Get up for the day!	Sleep-In Sunday
9.30am	Community meeting	Learning Centre	Learning Centre	Learning Centre	Learning Centre or Excursion (alternating weeks)	Breakfast Making Group	
11.00am	MORNING TEA	MORNING TEA	MORNING TEA	MORNING TEA		Activities with OT or Family Time	Activities with Nursing Staff or Family Time
11.20am	Learning Centre	Learning Centre	Music Therapy	Learning Centre			
12.30pm	LUNCH	LUNCH	LUNCH	LUNCH	LUNCH	LUNCH	LUNCH
1.00pm	Walking Group	Walking Group	Walking Group	Walking Group	Walking Group	Free time or Family time	Free time or Family time
1.30pm	Art Psychotherapy Group ©	What's The Feeling Group ©	Learning Centre	Peer Support Group	Open Art Studio		
2.30pm	AFTERNOON TEA	AFTERNOON TEA	AFTERNOON TEA	AFTERNOON TEA	AFTERNOON TEA	AFTERNOON TEA	AFTERNOON TEA
3.00pm	Sports group	Play Therapy Group	Teenage Life ©	Sensory Group	Music Therapy	Activities with Nursing Staff or Family Time	Open Art Studio with Nursing Staff
4.00pm	Activities with Nursing Staff or Family Time	Activities with Nursing Staff or Family Time	Master Chef	Sports group	Activities with Nursing Staff or Family Time		
5.30pm	DINNER	DINNER	DINNER	DINNER	DINNER	DINNER	DINNER
6.00pm	Homework/Free Time	Homework/Free Time	Pyjama Night	Board Games	Homework/Free Time	Homework/Free Time	Homework/Free Time
8.00pm	SUPPER	SUPPER	SUPPER	SUPPER	SUPPER	SUPPER	SUPPER
9.00pm	Wind down time (Electronics switched off) Music O.K.	Wind down time (Electronics switched off) Music O.K.	Wind down time (Electronics switched off) Music O.K.	Wind down time (Electronics switched off) Music O.K.	Wind down time (Electronics switched off) Music O.K.	Wind down time (Electronics switched off) Music O.K.	Wind down time (Electronics switched off) Music O.K.
9.30pm	BEDTIME	BEDTIME	BEDTIME	BEDTIME	BEDTIME	BEDTIME	BEDTIME

PLEASE NOTE: - From Monday to Friday, time with family (on or off the unit) occurs after all groups have finished, unless under special circumstances.
© - Indicates a closed group. Please check with facilitator beforehand.

Fig. 9.1 Timetable for the Walker Unit Group Therapy Programme. The programme is displayed in the living area of the ward and includes visuals which give an indication of the group content and the names of the staff who will run it

5. The 'Music Therapy Group' assists young people to play musical instruments as a non-verbal way of self-expression and this is facilitated by a registered music therapist (see Chap. 12).

6. The 'Teenage Life Group' is a space to explore common teenage experiences such as changes to friendship groups, puberty, experimentation, sexuality, peer pressure, schooling, drugs and alcohol, and family/carer dynamics. We find the young people who come to the Walker Unit have typically missed opportunities to learn about or discuss these matters owing to disengagement from school, youth groups, and peers. The aim of 'Teenage Life' is to create a safe space whereby young people can hear about experiences which may be the same or different to their own, creating a sense of camaraderie and a greater awareness and empathy for others. It is also a space to provide education on the above topics which young people may otherwise have difficulty accessing reliable information on. Examples include sexuality and recreational drug use. The group is currently facilitated by a speech pathologist and a clinical psychologist.

7. The 'Masterchef Group' is a cooking group facilitated by the occupational therapist. It is designed to support the young people to develop basic cooking skills in a social environment (see Chap. 13).

8. The 'Sensory Group' encourages awareness and experience of tactile, olfactory, auditory, gustatory, and visual sensory input through creating sensory items (see Figure 9.2) and sensory interventions, such as making aroma room spray, creating slime and play dough, practicing mindfulness, and using body movements like ball games and stretches. The sensory group is facilitated by the clinical psychologist and occupational therapist.

9. The 'Open Studio' group is designed to facilitate creative expression through the use of clay and art materials for enjoyment purposes, and to support young people to self-sooth in a relaxed and low stimulus environment. At times more embodied images may be expressed which are verbally acknowledged as a form of communication by the facilitator, and then referred back to the art therapist for appropriate follow up. It is facilitated by social work and psychology.

10. The 'Group Outing' is designed to support the young people to learn and practice their skills while "exposed" in the community. Skills include maintaining appropriate social behavior, budgeting, purchasing meals or tickets, participating in an age appropriate

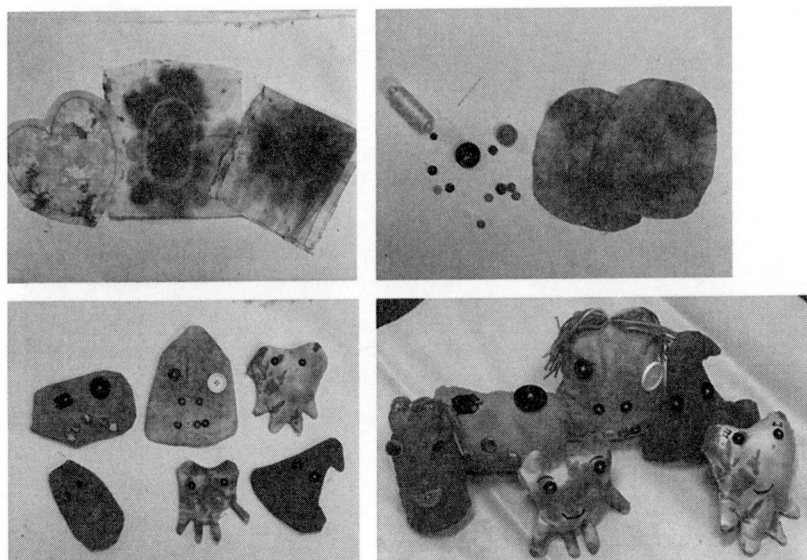

Fig. 9.2 Stages in the development of sensory items created by the young people

social activity. The group outing happens every second Friday morning and is facilitated by the occupational therapist and nursing staff.

11. The 'Walking Group' occurs after lunch and this is facilitated by the allied health and nursing team. It is usually a 30-minute walk around the hospital grounds and the aim is to encourage fresh air and exercise while practicing being off the ward as a group.

Some of the Challenges in Group Work

Chaos and ambivalence are often apparent in the group dynamics. Loud or playful interactions can turn into disruptive or unsafe behavior very quickly. For this reason, the group facilitators require expertise and clinical skills to manage the group safely, allowing the young person to practice riding this emotional wave with support and understanding. Therefore, the group therapy programme has an intention to allow tensions and distress to occur, so the young people may practice regulating their emotions and behavior.

Usually we have four allied health members working each weekday to ensure that group therapy, family therapy, and individual therapy progress safely. Due to the unpredictability of the young people, there are a variety of ways groups are delivered. For example, alternating non-verbal or verbal groups and the use of therapeutic spaces, such as courtyards or therapy rooms. Spontaneity, flexibility, and playful interactions are encouraged, with a tight frame held around the space for safety. For example, it can be helpful to think about appointments with medical staff, large families, or visiting clinicians during group therapy time to ensure that the group therapy programme does not get hijacked or forgotten.

Evenings and weekends are vulnerable times because the unit is staffed only by nurses. Handover from group facilitators to nursing staff regarding issues arising from group therapy session are essential. Weekend allied health support has also been helpful in the development of the group therapy programme. There is occupational therapy support available on Saturdays for an early breakfast or outing group (see Chap. 13). On Sundays, there is an art open studio group run by the nursing staff with assistance and follow up from the art therapist. This is further supported by ongoing in-servicing to the nursing staff. There has also been a baking group introduced late Sunday afternoons, for times when the young people had difficulty returning to the unit after leave. This would create a nurturing ambience across the ward from the smell of cake in the oven. We have found this intervention most helpful for those young people who might become aggressive when distressed.

Maintaining Therapeutic Gains from the Group Programme

In addition to some of the physical skills the young people gain from these group experiences, corrective emotional responses have been an important outcome and they are more likely to happen in the context of the group. Where some young people may have limitations, input by others can help working through difficult issues. The school room, group therapies, and family therapy meetings all offer opportunities for the young people to practice distress tolerance and emotional regulation. Expanding their window of tolerance and developing their contact with peers both on the ward and in their transition to community is an integrative process at the Walker Unit. Supporting them to re-attach to their peer community, usually at school or through another learning programme is crucial. The group therapy programme is a core foundation to the Walker admission.

References

Bo, S., Sharp, C., Beck, E., Pedersen, J., Gondan, M., & Simonsen, E. (2017). First empirical evaluation of outcomes for mentalization-based group therapy for adolescents with BPD. *Personal Disord, 8*(4), 396–401. https://doi.org/10.1037/per0000210

Chapman, L. (2014). *Neurobiology informed trauma therapy with children and adolescents. Understanding mechanisms of change.* Norton & Co.

Cozolino, J. L. (2002). *The neuroscience of psychotherapy: Building and rebuilding the human brain.* Norton & Co.

Garrick, D., & Ewashen, C. (2001). An integrated model for adolescent inpatient group therapy. *Journal of Psychiatric and Mental Health Nursing, 8*(2), 165–171. https://doi.org/10.1046/j.1365-2850.2001.00374.x

Griffith, D. (2010). Structure and containment in an adolescent inpatient acute unit and its groups. In J. Radcliffe, K. Hajek, J. Carson, & O. Manor (Eds.), *Psychological groupwork with acute psychiatric inpatients* (pp. 308–324). Whiting & Birch Ltd.

Gudiño, O. G., Weis, J. R., Havens, J. F., Biggs, E. A., Diamond, U. N., Marr, M., Jackson, C., & Cloitre, M. (2014). Group trauma-informed treatment for adolescent psychiatric inpatients: A preliminary uncontrolled trial. *Journal of Traumatic Stress, 27*(4), 496–500. https://doi.org/10.1002/jts.21928

Rippa, B. (2016). I am part of the group matrix. In S. S. Fehr (Ed.), *101 Interventions in group therapy* (pp. 265–268). Routledge.

Van der Kolk, B. A. (2015). *The body keeps the score: Brain, mind, and the body in the healing of trauma.* Penguin Group.

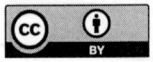

CHAPTER 10

Individual Psychotherapy

Tharushi Kaluarachchi, Karen Sarmiento, Matt Modini,
and Nina Mather

Abstract Adolescents admitted to the Walker Unit often present with complex mental health issues that have not responded well to previous treatment. Therefore, treatment at the Walker Unit requires flexibility within standard treatment approaches. This includes finding creative ways of building rapport, exploring difficult themes and negotiating achievable goals. The organisational set-up of the unit allows for increased frequency and flexibility with therapy sessions. Clinicians who deliver individual psychotherapy may also interact with the young person in other roles on the unit, which challenges the traditional notion of a singular patient-therapist relationship. In this chapter, we explore specific aspects of delivering psychotherapy to a severely unwell patient population.

T. Kaluarachchi (✉) • K. Sarmiento • M. Modini • N. Mather
Walker Unit, Concord Centre for Mental Health, Concord,
NSW, Australia
e-mail: Tharushi.Kaluarachchi@health.nsw.gov.au;
Karen.Sarmiento@health.nsw.gov.au;
matthew.modini@health.nsw.gov.au; Nina.Mather@health.nsw.gov.au

© The Author(s) 2022
P. Hazell (ed.), *Longer-Term Psychiatric Inpatient Care for
Adolescents*, https://doi.org/10.1007/978-981-19-1950-3_10

Keywords Adolescent • Inpatients • Mental health • Psychotherapy •
Cognitive behavioural therapy • Dialectical behaviour therapy

How Psychotherapy Looks at the Walker Unit

There is a growing number of evidence-based psychotherapies directed to treating psychopathology in adolescents (Gálvez-Lara et al., 2018). Evidence for psychotherapy has been gathered almost exclusively from studies of young people experiencing mild to moderately severe problems, with treatment being highly structured, short term and typically delivered in the community (Bettmann & Jasperson, 2009). It is uncertain whether findings gathered from such studies generalise to the inpatient setting. While the Walker Unit programme aims to deliver structured therapies such as dialectical behaviour therapy (DBT) and cognitive behavioural therapy (CBT), the severity of the psychiatric illness and the complexity of their relational and developmental issues means that young people may not have the capacity to engage with such treatment. Therapy usually needs to be delivered in a more flexible manner, tailored to the young person's particular difficulties and capacities.

Allocation of Therapist

Psychotherapy is delivered by allied health clinicians or psychiatry registrars alongside other therapeutic and rehabilitative components of the programme. In addition to a severe psychiatric illness, most young people admitted to the programme have experienced relational and attachment difficulties. Many have a history of complex trauma. There is thoughtful deliberation of the young person's needs, and their cognitive and verbal capacity to engage in psychotherapy. Additionally, consideration is given to the different approaches and therapeutic modalities which are used depending upon the therapist's orientation, training and strengths. Case examples are presented in Box 10.1 to illustrate these principles.

Box 10.1   Examples of Allocation to Individual Psychotherapy

Holly, a 15-year-old female, presented to the Walker Unit with a history of recurrent suicidal/self-harm behaviour, complex trauma, interpersonal difficulties, severe emotional dysregulation and eating issues. Holly had numerous acute inpatient admissions and interventions in the community with limited progress, often disengaging from clinicians. While deemed to have the capacity to engage she was largely disengaged and non-verbal in sessions. Given Holly's cognitive capacity and potential to engage verbally, she was assigned to a therapist with experience in dialectical behaviour therapy and working with young people with trauma.

Damien, a 17-year-old male, presented to the Walker Unit with obsessive compulsive disorder, autism spectrum disorder, odd posturing and movement, largely non-verbal, engaging in self-harm and at times displaying physically aggressive behaviours towards others. Damien was assigned to a therapist with experience treating obsessive compulsive disorder. However due to his other difficulties, Damien was also initially assigned to work with the speech pathologist to improve his communication skills.

Lily, a 16-year-old female, presented with social anxiety, depression, and attachment issues, a history of trauma and recurrent suicidal behaviour. She had multiple past short-stay inpatient admissions. Lily had fair engagement with past therapists and was motivated to attend the Walker Unit with the aim of resuming her engagement in schooling and the community. Lily was assigned to a therapist with experience in treating anxiety and depression and working with young people with a history of trauma.

Scheduling of Sessions

As in community care, young people have fixed appointment times for therapy. The frequency may be once or twice weekly, determined by need. This is typically decided in collaboration with the young person and accounts for factors such as; the capacity to engage and keep the focus of attention, the need for skill building sessions and time-limiting factors when the young person has increased home leave or is integrating to the home school. For a young person who has substantial difficulty tolerating therapy sessions or has a limited attention span, more frequent, brief sessions are indicated. If a young person refuses to attend a session, the therapist maintains the therapeutic frame by waiting in the therapy room for the allocated time and reflecting on the patient and their needs. The therapist then attempts to prompt the young person to reflect on their non-attendance.

Outside of scheduled sessions, the therapist may be called upon to provide support to the young person, usually in the context of them becoming distressed leading to self-harm or aggressive behaviour. After such an occurrence, the therapist might be involved in the chain analysis of the event. The information gained from the chain analysis can be used to prevent future escalation or help with early de-escalation when the early warning signs are recognised.

Working Within the Multidisciplinary Team

The individual therapist works alongside other members of the patient's multidisciplinary team including medical, nursing, education and other allied health staff. Clinicians will feedback on the process and content of individual sessions to team members as deemed appropriate and necessary for their treatment. This involves handing over key themes and processes of their internal world, reporting on therapeutic progress as well as other aspects relevant to their treatment such as their safety and interpersonal relationships. The information that is shared is integrated into their treatment by the whole treating team through discussions with the young person and their family, and helps to inform treatment decisions such as leave off the ward.

The therapist may also support other staff to better understand the emotional needs of a patient engaged in challenging behaviour. This can involve facilitating increased understanding regarding what is being communicated via the difficult behaviour and how staff may be able to respond therapeutically. In addition to formal meetings, therapists often find informal opportunities to discuss treatment with other team members. There is a delicate balance between sharing sufficient information with the multidisciplinary team to aid understanding, and maintaining the young person's confidentiality and right to privacy. The therapist will seek the young person's consent before disclosing to the multidisciplinary team sensitive material that has arisen in therapy.

Aspects of the Walker Unit that Facilitate Psychotherapy

Protected Environment

There is a high dropout rate amongst adolescent attending outpatient delivered psychotherapy. (Block & Greeno, 2011). In acute inpatient settings, psychotherapy is directed to crisis resolution. Patients admitted to the Walker Unit are provided with a longer admission, which facilitates more intensive treatment. The physical environment and the staffing on the ward allow for greater containment of risk of self-harm and suicide, factors which can severely disrupt treatment delivered in the community. The therapist is able to implement treatment that is potentially destabilising in the short term at the Walker Unit, as the secure environment provides a safety net for when patients respond adversely to issues that arise within their therapy. This may relate to uncovering distressing material, trauma-related work, more in-depth work on underlying emotional issues and entrenched belief systems or even challenging their attitudes and behaviour.

Protected Therapy Space

At the Walker Unit, the young person is provided with a separate therapy space, as their therapist is not involved in undertaking the family work. Given the wider family and systemic issues are part of the young person's pathology, maintaining this therapeutic boundary helps to foster trust and rapport. This increases the likelihood of the young person engaging with the clinician, being more receptive to discussing issues that may later be dealt with in the family therapy space.

Therapeutic Alliance

The therapeutic relationship, coupled with the therapeutic modality, characteristics of the young person and the therapist is known to make substantial contributions to the effectiveness of individual psychotherapy (Karver et al., 2018). The therapeutic relationship needs to foster a sense of trust, safety, containment and authenticity for the young person (Shirk et al., 2011). Most young people admitted to the Walker Unit have been exposed to multiple treatments with limited success. Some may have experienced breaches of trust in past therapies. While this presents an added challenge, the therapeutic relationship can be used to work through rejection, hostility and ambivalent dependence on the therapist. In the event that a therapeutic rupture takes place, the Walker setting and admission duration facilitates these formal and informal interactions for reparative work to take place.

Flexibility and Creativity

The nature of the Walker Unit treatment programme enables clinicians to be flexible and creative in overcoming barriers to treatment such as low motivation to engage in treatment, mistrust, hopelessness, severe emotional dysregulation, self-harming and aggressive behaviours and cognitive deficits. This can involve different tools of engagement such as playing games, making puzzles, using sensory toys, working on a shared activity, having sessions outside of the therapy room, for example, courtyard, going for a walk around the adjacent parklands. This reduces the expectation for verbal engagement, allows a point of focus in session and works on building tolerance to being in therapy.

The inpatient environment also allows clinicians frequent opportunities to work with issues that arise in the 'here and now', work on practising distress tolerance skills, engage in problem solving and chain analysis, which can ultimately teach better long-term coping skills. For example, a young person can be guided in the moment about working through these difficulties when incidents occur on the ward. Young people also work through a chain analysis after incidents have occurred with the therapist to identify underlying vulnerabilities, the situation and their internal world with the aim to reflect on their actions and improve upon this next time they feel distressed.

CHALLENGES TO DELIVERING PSYCHOTHERAPY AT THE WALKER UNIT

Poor Engagement

During individual therapy, the young person is encouraged to engage actively in their treatment. If capable, they may cite goals such as a reduction in symptoms, and achieving a more stable emotional state. However, this is often a very difficult task for young people who have had a large amount of therapeutic input in their lives and experience a sense of failure, hopelessness, and perceive a lack of capability in working towards their recovery. It is common for young people at the Walker Unit to be resistant to exploring difficult themes that emerge in psychotherapy. Owing to the level of treatment resistance and perceived hopelessness, unfortunately the therapy process may at times be directed more by the therapist, rather than being led by the patient. This lack of collaboration and investment in therapy can also mean that the rate of therapeutic progress with the young person is very slow.

Transference

For severely unwell young people, the delicate interaction between individual psychotherapy and other therapeutic elements in an inpatient unit can provide a recipe for developing strong transference reactions (Tsiantis, 1996). At the Walker Unit, the young person's level of symptomology, relational issues and the intensive nature of treatment can mean that transference themes which are challenging to manage emerge during the long-term admission. Therapists also need to be mindful of strong counter transference reactions towards patients which can compromise therapeutic care. The therapist then aims to use these reactions for therapeutic purposes, for example, responding non-defensively to a young person's hostility in the face of themes of abandonment and rejection and maintaining a consistent therapeutic framework. Clinicians manage this through regular supervision and therapeutic reflection with other team members to prevent this compromising the therapeutic care.

Multiple Roles

At the Walker Unit, no clinician exclusively interacts with a patient in the psychotherapy modality. Rather, therapists are involved in multiple roles with the young person, such as facilitating group therapies, group walks and outings, participating in community meeting, presenting MDT care plans, informal conversations and activities, at different points in the day. In each role, the clinician is actively engaging in different patterns of interaction with the young person. It can be advantageous in allowing the therapist to observe, engage and gain traction with the young person in their treatment in different settings and situations, particularly if the young person finds a certain aspect of their treatment difficult. The informal therapeutic spaces can also strengthen the relationship and provide opportunities for therapists to act in role-modelling healthy interactions. However, while the therapist will gain more exposure to the young person, the therapist needs to be mindful of respecting the boundaries between therapeutic interactions. While generally therapists will stick to strict codes of non-self-disclosure, often at the Walker Unit, given the lengthy admission, therapists are not able to be as rigid in their therapeutic role. They will carefully navigate these boundaries and may self-disclose personal information on casual topics if this is deemed beneficial for the patient. As clinicians hold a delicate therapeutic relationship with the young person, they need to be mindful of the impact of the different roles on each other and despite the fluidity of the roles attempt to maintain a sense of consistency. If issues arise, it should be specifically addressed with the young person to repair the relationship and discussed with the wider treating team.

CONCLUSION

Psychotherapy at the Walker Unit calls on finding flexibility and creativity in delivering evidence-based treatments, with an emphasis on working with a protected individual space and within a multidisciplinary team approach to tackle treatment difficulties and engage severely unwell young people. Generally, challenges are encountered in juggling multiple clinical roles, while managing poor engagement and transference reactions that occur in the longer term setting. While these challenges occur, ultimately it is very rewarding and provides a unique opportunity for this intensive treatment to be delivered in a vulnerable population.

REFERENCES

Bettmann, J. E., & Jasperson, R. A. (2009). Adolescents in residential and inpatient treatment: A review of the outcome literature. *Child & Youth Care Forum, 38*(4), 161–183.

Block, A. M., & Greeno, C. G. (2011). Examining outpatient treatment dropout in adolescents: A literature review. *Child and Adolescent Social Work Journal, 28*(5), 393–420.

Gálvez-Lara, M., Corpas, J., Moreno, E., Venceslá, J. F., Sánchez-Raya, A., & Moriana, J. A. (2018). Psychological treatments for mental disorders in children and adolescents: A review of the evidence of leading international organizations.

Clinical Child and Family Psychology Review, 21(3), 366–387. https://doi. org/10.1007/s10567-018-0257-6

Karver, M. S., De Nadai, A. S., Monahan, M., & Shirk, S. R. (2018). Meta-analysis of the prospective relation between alliance and outcome in child and adolescent psychotherapy. *Psychotherapy (Chicago, Ill.), 55*(4), 341–355. https://doi. org/10.1037/pst0000176

Shirk, S. R., Karver, M. S., & Brown, R. (2011). The alliance in child and adolescent psychotherapy. *Psychotherapy (Chicago, Ill.), 48*(1), 17–24. https://doi. org/10.1037/a0022181

Tsiantis, J. (1996). Transference and countertransference issues in the in-patient psychotherapy of traumatized children and adolescents. In A.-M. S. J. Tsiantis, D. Anastasopoulos, & B. Martindale (Eds.), *Countertransference in psychoanalytic psychotherapy with children and adolescents*. International Universities Press.

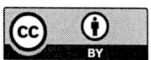

CHAPTER 11

Art Therapy

Fran Nielsen

Abstract The use of group art therapy, individual art therapy and family art therapy in an inpatient child and adolescent mental health services unit will be described, including images and consumer feedback to demonstrate effectiveness. The artworks made in art therapy can reveal hidden dysfunction in the young person and/or their family members. Recent trauma research supports capacity to access this material safely through non-verbal visual communication. Family art therapy has been a useful intervention to support the identification of illness in a parent, to improving attunement between the parent and the child and for the parent to detach from their child's symptoms by agreeing to get treatment for themselves. If the patient cannot separate from the illness in the parent, their symptoms will persist.

Keywords Adolescent • Inpatients • Mental Health • Art Therapy

---

The original version of this chapter was revised. The correction to this chapter can be found at https://doi.org/10.1007/978-981-19-1950-3_21

F. Nielsen (✉)
Walker Unit, Concord Centre for Mental Health, Concord, NSW, Australia
e-mail: Fran.Nielsen@health.nsw.gov.au

95

What the Art Therapy is Doing at the Walker Unit

Art Therapy is an emerging practice in mental health settings, particularly for children and families who experience trauma induced symptoms (Kozlowska & Hanney, 1999; Nielsen et al., 2019). Many of the young people and their family members experience verbal communication difficulties. Where previous standard interventions have been ineffective, they often enter the unit anxious and fatigued. The art therapist in this unit provides structured individual, family and group-based art therapy treatment by working non-verbally with art materials as part of care. The non-verbal approach of art therapy has been effective in engaging this difficult to treat group of young people (Nielsen, 2018; Nielsen et al., 2019, 2021).

While most psychological therapy interventions inform the framework for art therapy, in this setting there has been an opportunity to further develop a "responsive art psychotherapy" practice (Havsteen-Franklin, 2014; Nielsen, 2018). The art therapist has been able to contain emotionally charged projected experiences, by their capacity to provide an interpretive visual response in session. This has been particularly helpful when the young person or their family member is in the early phases of treatment and are unable to reflect upon, or make any links between their thoughts, feelings and behaviours.

Working on the young person's willingness to engage is a common first line goal in treatment. By their engagement with the art therapy in the group programme, the young people have an opportunity to express their distress safely, using art materials to develop an understanding of containing difficult emotions for themselves. During the group programme, it has been important for the art therapist to facilitate their safety in this experience by participating in the art making process alongside the young people. Depending on the capacities of the young people, after the artmaking, a discussion may occur. They are invited to look and think about the artworks made in the group process. For those unable to reflect, individual art therapy may be recommended. This is especially helpful if themes of trauma are emerging in the artworks. Supporting them with their capacity to communicate difficult internal experiences safely is the focus of the art therapy. Then by looking at what has been represented in the artworks, over time they are able to sit with and think more about what has been externalised in the object of the artworks made.

As many of the young people and their families experience verbal communication difficulties, art therapy can safely assist the young person and/

or family member to non-verbally communicate their feelings at a pace that is comfortable for them and support their thinking (or more accurately incapacity to think), grounding them in the present and feelings of safety. As the young person and/or family member engages in their art-making, by making a response artwork an experienced senior art therapist can non-verbally support the unintegrated fragments of their emotionally overwhelmed experience. The sensory movements involved in artmaking seem to enable access to dissociated experiences safely (Chong, 2015). The implicit non-verbal communications made in the artworks can be a useful contribution in treatment, as trauma content can be revealed in images long before the cognition and explicit narrative is available (Bucci, 2007a; Nielsen, 2018).

Working with dissociation safely in the art therapy has been a main component of in-session practice at the Walker Unit. Recent trauma research supports capacity to access this material safely through non-verbal visual communication (Coulter, 2015; Hoshino & Cameron, 2008; Nielsen, 2018). The main goal of the art therapy in this setting is to stabilise emotional dysregulation and increase tolerance for distress. In some cases, the family members may present as distressed as the young person. As a right brain to right brain non-verbal activity, artmaking alongside the family member and the young person has had the potential to evoke the curative factor of a shared dysregulated to regulated experience (Nielsen et al., 2021; Schore, 2011). This has given these young people and their families hope for agency and change, despite the losses in their capacities to verbally communicate their feelings. The images in Fig. 11.1 demonstrate how an art therapist might make a non-verbal response (right) in the containment of the young person's distress (represented in the images on the left).

How the Art Therapy is Implemented at the Walker Unit

All art therapy, individual, group and family sessions are structured and planned with the multi-disciplinary team. When the art therapy is introduced to the young person and/or family member, there is a common anxiety for those unfamiliar to the materials to think that art skills are required. Often an art therapist will begin by explaining this is not the case and that the main requirement is to 'have a go.' This can get under the

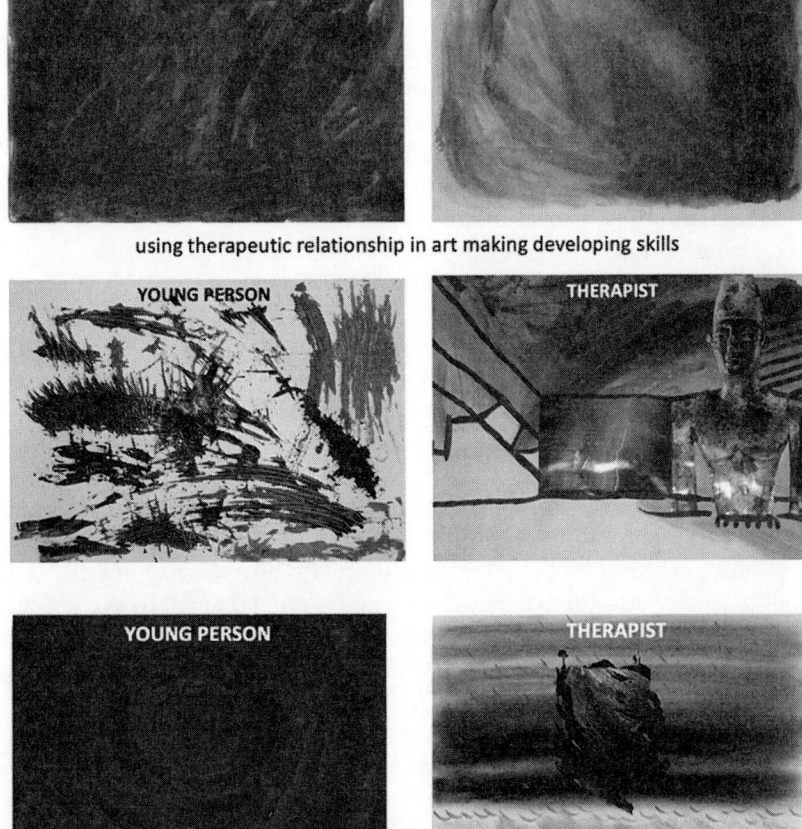

Fig. 11.1 Young person and therapist images

wire of the reluctance to engage and appeal to their capacity to play, experiment or explore new ideas. To make a mark on the paper is the only requirement. Boundaries within the art room are explained, for example, not talking about other people's work in the art room and that there is a locked art therapy cupboard provided for storage and safety of the artworks made. This is an important intervention to ensure the safety and containment of the shared internal experiences made explicit by the artworks.

Three assessment sessions are often introduced when there is a referral and after the third session, a summary is shared including images, to reflect on the young person or family member's availability to engage and think about their work. After producing at least three artworks, an art therapy consent form is signed by the young person and/or family member for the permission to photograph or share images and include them in MDT meetings, art therapy reports, educational in-services and/or research publications. Some of the principles and procedures within art therapy practice are shared. This can encourage collaboration from the young person or family member regarding their ongoing engagement, responsibilities and capacity to think about what is happening for themselves.

Images can be utilised as documents to their experience. They are able to demonstrate capacity for change or cognition to function and can offer information beyond text by measuring "intonation, gesture, tempo." (Sagan, 2019). Symbols can be another measure of a patient's developing capacity to communicate, by non-verbally, bringing what was implicit into explicit conscious form (Bucci, 2007a, 2007b). Examples of the non-verbal shift from implicit, dissociative content to the more explicit symbolic content are presented in Fig. 11.2.

 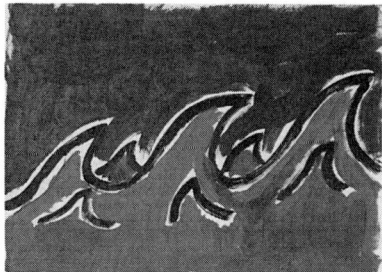

Images from raw dissociative experiences (left) to symbolic form (right)

 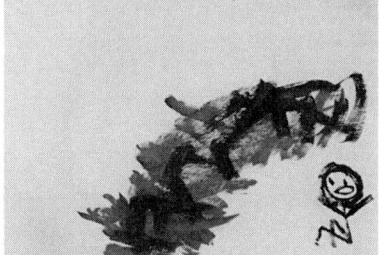

Fig. 11.2 Shift from dissociative to symbolic content

When words are in the work the cognition is more likely to function alongside the difficult feeling (Fig. 11.3).

The sequence in Fig. 11.4 demonstrates the layers and detail of how an embodied image can be made and is an example of what cannot be thought about or put into words by the young person or family member.

Where diagrammatic content is applied to the embodied feeling, consciousness and thought forms are made available to the young person or family member. Symbolic examples in Fig. 11.5 demonstrate line and form emerging in the imagery and demonstrate a capacity for integration of thoughts and feelings.

When the young person is feeling distressed with thoughts of suicide or self-harm and makes images such as Fig. 11.5, it is more possible for them to safely integrate their feelings, strengthening their 'emotional muscle' and building their confidence and competencies to survive the thoughts for a safer outcome.

When the young person is experiencing psychosis, it is almost impossible for them to integrate their thoughts and feelings, their internal experience may remain fragmented and detached. Art as therapy can provide an option for the young people to self sooth or distract themselves, as in Fig. 11.6.

The images in Fig. 11.7 reflect a young person who was floridly psychotic, after some time in silence they had said, "I have all these thoughts

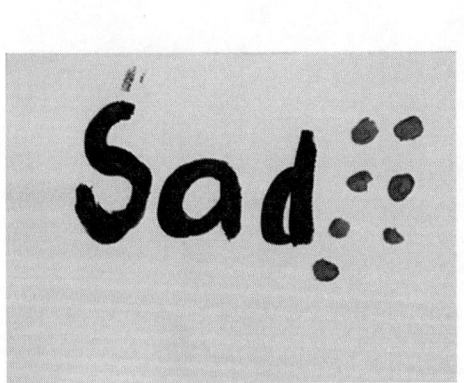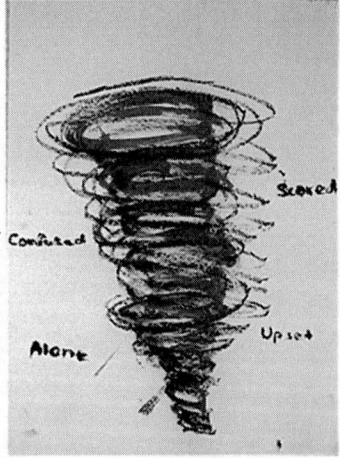

Fig. 11.3 Words in artwork

Fig. 11.4 Embodied image

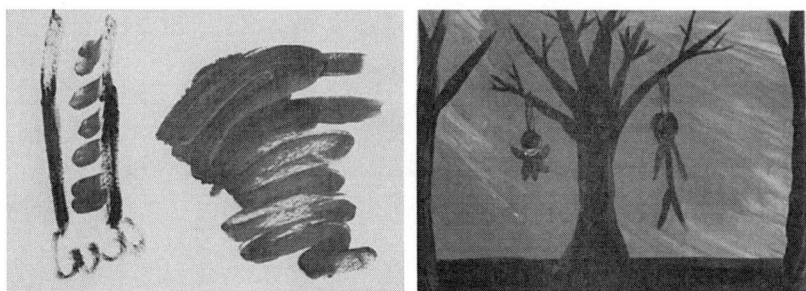

Fig. 11.5 Integration of feelings

I don't know where they come from and they make me say things I don't want to say." The image has, "I am a train" scratched into it. Such images can assist with reality checking.

Figure 11.8 outlines a generalised process for the art therapy treatment at the Walker Unit

Fig. 11.6 Art for
soothing and distraction

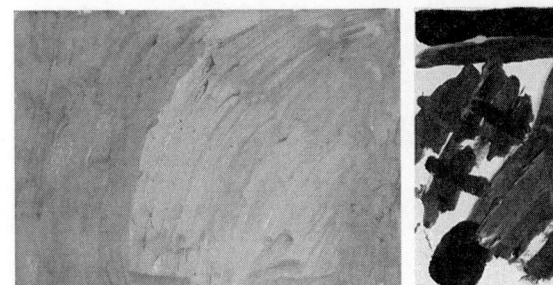

Fig. 11.7 Psychotic images

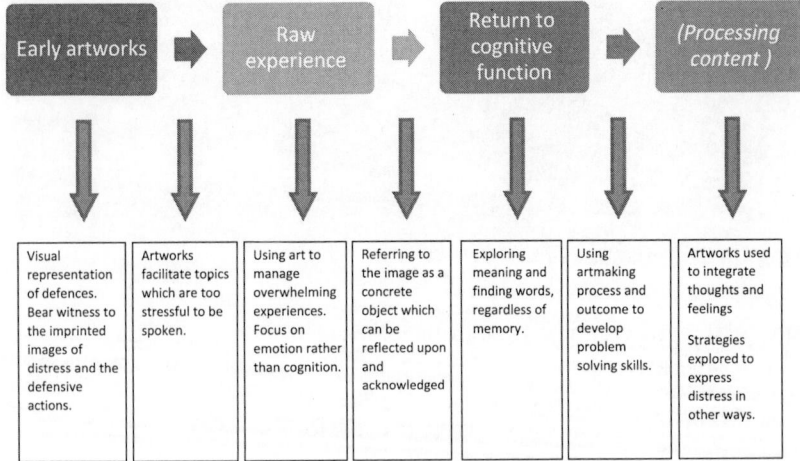

Early artworks	Raw experience	Return to cognitive function	(Processing content)

Visual representation of defences. Bear witness to the imprinted images of distress and the defensive actions.	Artworks facilitate topics which are too stressful to be spoken.	Using art to manage overwhelming experiences. Focus on emotion rather than cognition.	Referring to the image as a concrete object which can be reflected upon and acknowledged	Exploring meaning and finding words, regardless of memory.	Using artmaking process and outcome to develop problem solving skills.	Artworks used to integrate thoughts and feelings Strategies explored to express distress in other ways.

Fig. 11.8 The process of art therapy

The Art Therapy Space

The art therapy room is located opposite the seclusion room which is rare for an art room as they are usually located away from the main ward. The art therapy room has remained low stimulus and the walls neutral for the young person or family member to feel safe to enter. The palette of materials are limited and in 'good enough' condition. It is important for the young person to understand the art therapist is not there to entertain them. Neither is it a performance driven activity, as it might be in the school setting. Figure 11.9 identifies the materials used and how the table is set.

Outcomes

A data base of images as well as the young people's feedback has been gathered to demonstrate effectiveness (Nielsen et al., 2019). Eighty per cent of the young people at the Walker Unit have reported that art therapy has helped them to express themselves safely and begin to think about how their thoughts and feelings relate to their behaviours. Previously this had been difficult for

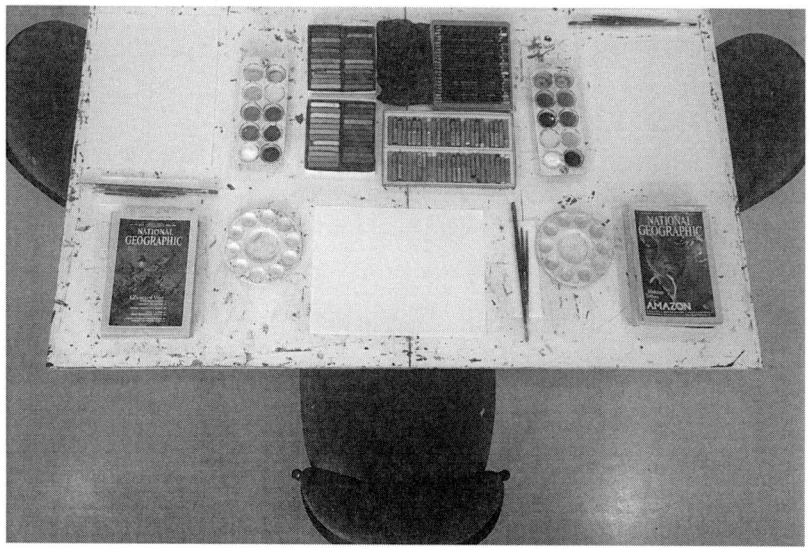

Fig. 11.9 Art materials

them to do. Families have also contributed to feedback and reported they have found art therapy to be helpful (Nielsen et al., 2021). The young people and sometimes family members also contribute to their art therapy reports by choosing their images and finding the words to communicate their experiences. This has been particularly important as a handover document for the young person to communicate their needs, as the verbal therapies remain standard practice in the community.

CONCLUSION AND RECOMMENDATIONS

Verbal interventions may be too challenging for young people or family members who feel unsafe with their thoughts and feelings. Supporting them with their capacity to communicate difficult internal experiences safely has been the focus of the art therapy at the Walker Unit with the main goal, to stabilise emotional dysregulation and increase tolerance for distress. Responsive art making (Havsteen-Franklin & Altamirano, 2015; Nielsen, 2018; Nielsen et al., 2019, 2021) is an emerging clinical practice within art therapy. This practice is used in this setting with the young people and their families and challenges common beliefs that the purpose of images is to solicit a narrative. There is a lack of awareness of the capacity for non-verbal visual art therapy experiences in mental health services. A permanent 32 hour a week position has made it possible for the art therapist in this setting to provide a consistent approach for the young people and their families, while maintaining flexibility with the team. This is very rare for art therapy practitioners and more positions need to be made available to support mental health services in the future. The permanency of the role has also supported research opportunities, an important consideration for the development of art therapy positions to be maintained in the future.

REFERENCES

Bucci, W. (2007a). Dissociation from the perspective of Multiple Code Theory—Part I. *Contemporary Psychoanalysis, 43*(2), 165–184.

Bucci, W. (2007b). Dissociation from the perspective of Multiple Code Theory—Part II. *Contemporary Psychoanalysis, 43*(3), 305–326.

Chong, C. (2015). Why art psychotherapy? Through the lens of interpersonal neurobiology: The distinctive role of art psychotherapy interventions for clients with early relational trauma. *International Journal of Art Therapy, 20*(3), 118–126.

Coulter, A. M. (2015). Family art therapy: Dots, meaning and metaphor. In C. Kerr (Ed.), *Multicultural family art therapy* (pp. 90–104). Routledge.

Havsteen-Franklin, D. (2014). Consensus for using an arts-based response in art therapy. *International Journal of Art Therapy, 19*(3), 107–113.

Havsteen-Franklin, D., & Altamirano, J. C. (2015). Containing the uncontainable: Responsive art making in art therapy as a method to facilitate mentalization. *International Journal of Art Therapy, 20*(2), 54–65.

Hoshino, J., & Cameron, C. (2008). Narrative art therapy within a multicultural framework. In C. Kerr (Ed.), *Family art therapy: Foundations of theory and practice.* Routledge.

Kozlowska, K., & Hanney, L. (1999). Family assessment and intervention using an interactive art exercise. *Australian & New Zealand Journal of Family Therapy, 20*(2), 61–69.

Nielsen, F. (2018). Responsive Art Psychotherapy as a component of intervention for severe adolescent mental illness: A case study. *Art Therapy OnLine (ATOL), 9*, 1–38.

Nielsen, F., Feijo, I., Renshall, K., & Starling, J. (2021). Family Art Therapy: A contribution to mental health treatment in an adolescent inpatient setting. *Australian and New Zealand Journal of Family Therapy., 42*, 145–159.

Nielsen, F., Isobel, S., & Starling, J. (2019). Evaluating the use of responsive art therapy in an inpatient child and adolescent mental health services unit. *Australasian Psychiatry, 27*(2), 165–170. https://doi.org/10.1177/1039856218822745

Sagan, O. (2019). Art-making and its interface with dissociative identity disorder: No words that didn't fit. *Journal of Creativity in Mental Health, 14*(1), 23–36.

Schore, A. N. (2011). The right brain implicit self lies at the core of psychoanalysis. *Psychoanalytic Dialogues, 21*, 75–100.

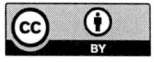

CHAPTER 12

Music Therapy

Joanne McIntyre

Abstract The Walker Unit is one of only a few adolescent inpatient units in Australia to include a Registered Music Therapist on the Allied Health team. The Walker Unit has a music room equipped with guitars, ukuleles, a keyboard, a drum kit, African drums, a cello and a violin. Music therapy sessions are conducted with individuals, patient groups and families. Empirical evidence supporting the benefits of Music Therapy in this setting is limited, however we have observed that creating music in a containing environment enhances self-awareness, stimulates verbalization and facilitates relaxation.

Keywords Adolescent • Inpatients • Mental Health • Music Therapy

Introduction

Music therapy has been part of the programme at the Walker Unit since October 2010. Group sessions, individual sessions and family sessions are available to patients during admission. This non-verbal, expressive

J. McIntyre (✉)
Peninsula Music Services, Sydney, NSW, Australia

© The Author(s) 2022
P. Hazell (ed.), *Longer-Term Psychiatric Inpatient Care for Adolescents*, https://doi.org/10.1007/978-981-19-1950-3_12

modality is often found to assist patients who find it difficult and challenging to put their experiences and feelings into words. Music therapy has been described as "well-suited" to the adolescent psychiatric inpatient unit as "the symbolic and structural nature of music provides adolescent inpatients with a unique framework in which both intrapersonal phenomena and interpersonal experiences can be expressed and explored" (Frisch, 1990). When the young person engages in music therapy, it may assist them to work through emotions arising from trauma they may have experienced, as well as assist them in their own growth and development. Erickson commented on music therapy as part of a hospital programme by saying, "This program has become an indispensable counterpart to psychotherapy, and has proven fertile in testing and promoting the inner resources of young people in acute crisis" (Erikson, 1968).

WHY MUSIC THERAPY AT THE WALKER UNIT?

The importance that music has in adolescents' everyday life is evidenced by the amount of music they listen to and the time they spend listening to it. Active music making, for example, playing a musical instrument, has benefits for adolescents. Group music therapy offers adolescents a secure and supportive environment in which to freely experiment with instruments and sounds, and to engage with others musically. Exposure to music making and active music listening when teamed together in a music therapy session, have been seen to display many positive benefits for participating adolescents. Research indicates that the importance of music and the use of music in a young person's day to day life does in fact correlate with their psychosocial development (Laiho, 2004) and therefore may be considered as an important ingredient in "enabling and empowering" adolescents (Cheong-Clinch, 2009).

GROUP MUSIC THERAPY

A twice-weekly group music therapy session gather the young people to engage in music making and to explore "musicking" in a therapeutic way. Each session is designed to encourage participants to discover and experiment with another way of expressing emotions by engaging in music both practically and through discussion. Each session has time for structured music making and for improvisation using musical instruments, based on each person's needs at the time.

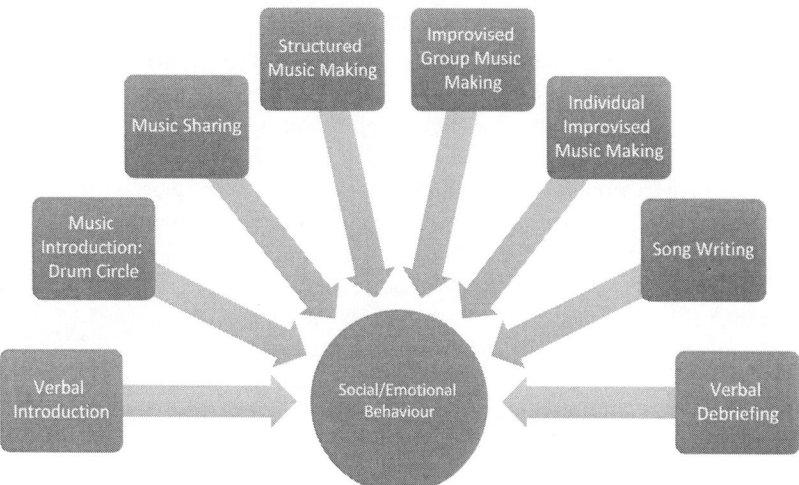

Fig. 12.1 Techniques used in music therapy

To assist in making playing music accessible for the patients, the Walker Unit purchased a number of musical instruments in 2011. The instruments purchased include an electric guitar, a bass guitar, two amplifiers, two acoustic guitars, a digital full-sized keyboard, a drum kit, African drums, a cello and a violin. Ukuleles are also used during sessions as often patients have their own ukulele with them.

What Happens in a Music Therapy Group Session?

Figure 12.1 illustrates the different techniques that may be employed in a music therapy session to assist with a young person's social/emotional behaviour.

Verbal Introduction

On entering the music therapy space, the therapist checks in with each participant to assess how they are feeling and what they have been doing since the last session. This may include conversation around what they did on leave, if they had any leave, weekend activities, family meeting discussion and if they have discovered any new music since the last session. It also assists in settling the patients so they can engage more easily in the music.

Music Introduction (Drum Circle)

After the verbal introduction, a music introduction to the session sets the mood and pace of the session. Each participant is given a djembe (African drum) and asked to follow the lead of the therapist. The therapist gives a very simple beat to play so each person can copy it. As the participants begin to play in time with each other, the therapist changes the rhythm. This simple change in rhythm can reveal who is listening, who is watching and who is rhythmical. From the moment the participants touch the drumheads, it becomes clear as to how the young person is going to respond to the music in the session. For example, a young person who is just lightly touching the drum with one finger and cannot be heard probably won't play much in the session. Someone who has a closed fist and punches the centre of the drum on the other hand, will probably dominate the volume of the session and may be difficult to contain.

Music Sharing

In addition to playing instruments, there is opportunity and encouragement to share pre-recorded music in the group. Music sharing is an effective way of gauging how the group is functioning as individuals and as a group. Encouraging young people to share what they have recently been listening to enables the therapist to assess mood, thought content and general connection with the young persons' world. It also assists with knowing what the young person is spending their time listening to and thinking about outside of the music therapy room. Issues such as emotions, identity, relationships and memories can be approached in song lyrics without the same confrontation as asking questions or seeking verbal interaction.

Discussion often develops from listening to pre-recorded songs and often the group members talk more freely when their own song is being played. The strong connection with song choice may prompt them to speak about issues or challenges that usually they may not share publicly with their peers or with a therapist. Song sharing also acts as a way to encourage group cohesion and interaction if the participants have arrived to the session unsettled.

Structured Music Making

Structured music making occurs when the therapist arranges a particular song or piece of music so each participant can play an instrument to create an interpretation of an already written song. Songs used for structured music making include popular songs known to the patients as well as classic hits from the past. There are some songs that work well with this age group and this can be made accessible for all stages of musical experience. These include "Radioactive", "When September Ends", "We Will Rock You", "Under The Bridge", "Riptide", "Imagine", "I'm Yours", "Smoke on The Water" and "It's a Long Way to the Top". These songs are easy to adapt and can be utilized with most levels of music training or experience.

The process of playing a musical instrument in structured music making can facilitate self-expression by projecting personal thoughts and feelings into the music being played. It may also enhance self-awareness, stimulate verbalization and provide a pleasurable, non-threatening environment for the group members. Playing together as a group can also facilitate relaxation, often with the end result of reducing tension and anxiety in the participant.

Improvised Group Music Making

The transition from structured to improvised music can be challenging. This is where the training of the RMT to support group improvisation becomes important. To assist with the group improvisation, the therapist can play a chord progression that fits in with the general tuning of the instruments being used. This then makes the sound of the instruments being played more tonal and easier for the players to listen to. A good example of this is when a cello is being played, a suitable chord progression would be in C Major. As the open strings of the cello are played, the chords played in C fit in and sound resonant with the cello. This then encourages the young person to play and improvise without sounding unpleasant to their ear.

The more familiar the group is with each other and with the therapist, the easier it becomes to explore the creative and expressive responses of each individual in improvisation. For some, improvisation is confronting.

For others, the energy and excitement of playing whatever they like with the group is something they enjoy doing and appear to benefit from, for example, in self-confidence and positive mood changes.

For some young people however, the nature of the issues surrounding their admission may cause a block in free creativity and improvisation. When this occurs, the therapist scaffolds the improvisation by using some structured music to gradually assist the young person to play and offers suggestions on what notes and techniques to use on their instrument. This has proven to assist some who have limited musical experience or who are experiencing challenging mental health issues that stop the flow of creativity.

Individual Improvised Music Making

During the group improvisation, the therapist invites each group member to play solo while the therapist supports on the keyboard. Soloing in the group improvisation is used as a way of encouraging each participant to play publicly as well as to play along with the therapist. Inviting the young person to the keyboard to co-improvise then further develops this style of improvisation. Not all group members are comfortable with individual improvisation at the keyboard, so not everyone is asked to do this. When the young person accepts the invitation to play, they sit at the treble end of the keyboard while the therapist sits at the bass end. The young person is then asked to play the keyboard with one or both hands, playing the white notes only. As they begin to play, the therapist joins them and supports what they are playing by adding chords, echoing melody and adding musical ideas. After the improvisation ends, the therapist then asks the group and the individual whether they were reminded of anything as the music was playing, or whether they felt an emotion. If anyone comments about what they experienced during the improvisation, it is further discussed and processed as a group.

Song Writing

Song writing with adolescents is an active way of gleaning information about their thoughts, hopes and aspirations as well as their fears and doubts. This activity can be facilitated in many different ways including

1. Word substitution with a known song
2. Using words from a poem written by a group member
3. Each member writing one line of lyrics and adding it to the group song
4. The therapist providing a poem to use as lyrics
5. Using a software package like Garage Band, Music Lab or Pro-Tools to make beats

Whatever method is chosen, the aim is to put thoughts, ideas and feelings into a song so they can be processed through a music lens. Song writing assists this process by being a more focused and permanent way of recording feelings and discussing them. When a song is completed, the therapist records the finished work and then plays it back to the group for further discussion.

Verbal Debriefing

Verbal debriefing at the end of the session can assist with supporting group members to process what they have just experienced in the group. The therapist asks each person to choose a member and find a positive comment to say about what the person played or contributed in the group session. This last part of the music therapy group can improve self-awareness each young person as they sit with positive comments being said about them.

THE FUTURE OF MUSIC THERAPY AT THE WALKER UNIT

At the time of writing, the registered music therapist working at the Walker Unit is contracted to work eight hours per week spread equally over two days. There is a plan to turn the contract position into a permanent part time position of between 8–16 hours. This is currently being written and once it has been approved, and a registered music therapist is employed, music therapy will have more stability and a greater contribution to the individual health plans of the young people admitted to the Walker inpatient programme.

REFERENCES

Cheong-Clinch, C. (2009). Music for engaging young people in education. *Youth Studies Australia, 28*, 50–57.

Erikson, E. (1968). *Identity, youth and crisis.* W. W Norton & Co., Inc.

Frisch, A. (1990). Symbol and structure: Music therapy for the adolescent psychiatric inpatient. *Music Therapy, 9*(1), 16–34.

Laiho, S. (2004). The psychological functions of music in adolescence. *Nordic Journal of Music Therapy, 13*(1), 47–63. https://doi.org/10.1080/08098130409478097

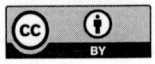

CHAPTER 13

Occupational Therapy

Polly Kwan

Abstract Occupational therapy aims to engage individuals in meaningful tasks to improve and maintain their performance and quality of life. At the Walker Unit, occupational therapists assist young people to increase their independence and overall mental wellbeing through practical daily activities in the home and community, and through sensory-based interventions. Sensory approaches facilitate self-regulation in regards to both physiological and emotional arousal. Young people with mental health problems also have unique sensory experiences and needs, which should be understood by clinicians and caregivers to promote a sensory supportive experience to aid their recovery. The Walker Unit has embraced the sensory framework, incorporating the use of sensory-based interventions into treatment and everyday living.

Keywords Adolescent • Inpatients • Mental health • Occupational therapy • Social participation

P. Kwan (✉)
Walker Unit, Concord Centre for Mental Health, Concord, NSW, Australia
e-mail: Polly.Kwan@health.nsw.gov.au

© The Author(s) 2022
P. Hazell (ed.), *Longer-Term Psychiatric Inpatient Care for Adolescents*, https://doi.org/10.1007/978-981-19-1950-3_13

What Does the Occupational Therapist at the Walker Unit Do Exactly?

Occupational therapy is a complex intervention with multiple interacting components that aims to engage individuals in meaningful tasks. The goals of occupational therapy are to improve and maintain quality of life and occupational performance in the area of self-care, productivity and leisure. In inpatient mental health settings, occupational therapists typically have a major role in leading the group therapy programme and providing vocational support (Fossey & Bramley, 2014). At the Walker Unit, the responsibility for running therapy groups is shared equally among the multidisciplinary team, while the Department of Education addresses the educational and vocational needs of the young people. This raises the question, what is the specific role of the occupational therapist in the Walker Unit programme?

As a member of the multidisciplinary team, occupational therapists at the Walker Unit have both a generic child and adolescent mental health professional role (i.e. providing individual therapy, group therapy and family therapy), and a specialist occupational therapist role, working with the young person across multiple domains. The specialised tasks of the occupational therapist are summarised in Fig. 13.1.

Occupational therapists at the Walker Unit are classified as a shift worker, with a mix of regular day, afternoon and weekend shifts. Most individual therapy sessions and clinical meetings usually occur during the day shift, while the afterhours shift affords the opportunity to engage and support the young people in other creative ways. For example, one evening each week the young people prepare and eat a meal under the supervision of the occupational therapist, after which they watch together an episode of the television series, "Master Chef". On the weekend, the occupational therapist may take one or more of the young people off the unit for an excursion. This is particularly helpful when a young person's family is unable to visit, as it provides an opportunity to shop for personal items. It also affords an opportunity for the young person to practice some of the skills listed below.

The goals of occupational therapy interventions include improving independence and the overall wellbeing of the young people through practical daily activities in their home and community. This typically involves supporting the young people to challenge themselves to gradually

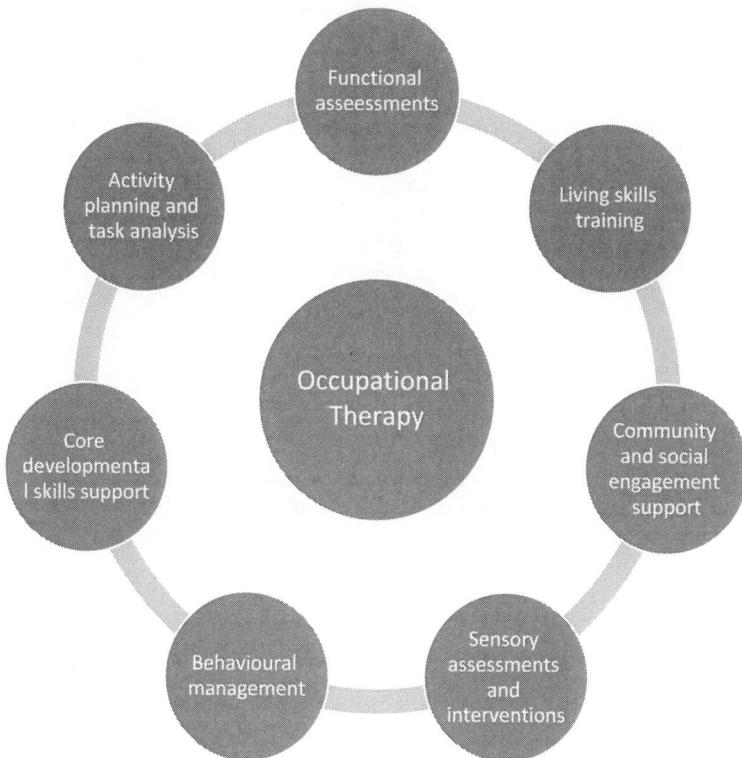

Fig. 13.1 Discipline—specific roles of the occupational therapist

expose and engage in a variety of daily activities, such as cooking, shopping, budgeting, catching public transport and self-care tasks. Young people with trauma experiences, attachment difficulties, neurodevelopmental disorders (e.g. autism spectrum disorder and attention deficit hyperactivity disorder) or mental illness (e.g. psychosis, anxiety and mood disorders) often have difficulties participating in these day-to-day living tasks or engaging in meaningful activities. The occupational therapist at the Walker Unit faces the challenges of safely engaging the young people in these daily activities in the context of a restrictive secure environment. The following case examples illustrate the role of the occupational therapist:

Anna, 16 years of age, was admitted to the Walker Unit to manage her suicidality and recurrent self-harm. She was anxious about returning to her parent's care after discharge, owing to a seemingly irreparable breakdown in family relationships. A supported accommodation placement was explored as an alternative discharge destination. Living in supported accommodation would require Anna to develop a repertoire of skills she had not needed while living with her parents. Knowing that the treating team supported her need to live away from home, Anna became more motivated to work on maintaining her safety. She was relatively independent with the basic activities of daily living, however she had not developed age appropriate skills. While living with her parents, Anna had restricted access to the kitchen and other places that might provide her with the means to self-harm. Clearly, if Anna was to live in supported accommodation where self-catering is common, she would need to demonstrate that she was safe in the kitchen environment. The occupational therapy interventions for Anna included assessing and monitoring her risks through different day-to-day activities; and providing training in these activities through graded exposure. Anna participated in the cooking group learning basic food preparation skills, and was exposed to a range of "risky" tools during different cooking tasks (e.g. the hot electric fry pan, the electrical cord from the toaster). She used safety scissors while engaging in craft activities. The tools selected for each activity were thoughtfully planned. Following a thorough risk assessment and discussion with the treating team, the occupational therapist began to work with Anna outside the Walker Unit, training her how to get to the shops by public transport, taking her along to the shops to buy ingredients for the cooking groups, helping her to set up a bank account and mobile phone plan, and developing a weekly budget plan with her.

Bella was a 15 years old girl who presented with psychosis and post-traumatic stress disorder symptoms. She was disorganised, with an associated decline in her functioning. She struggled with following the therapy program or attending to the basic activities of daily living. After discovering Bella's interest in baking, the occupational therapist decided to use cooking as an intervention to engage her in therapy. A daily routine checklist was created for Bella focusing on the basic activities of daily living, such as showering, dressing in clean clothes, and brushing teeth (Fig. 13.2). Classroom and group participation were also included in the checklist as per her treatment plan. Bella could earn individual baking time with the occupational therapist when she demonstrated an effort in attempting those tasks on the checklist. Selection of the recipes and the baking tools had to be carefully planned due to Bella's high aggression risk and low attention span. The occupational therapist assessed Bella's functioning level through the baking activity, (e.g. how she organised the ingredients, how she followed the steps from the

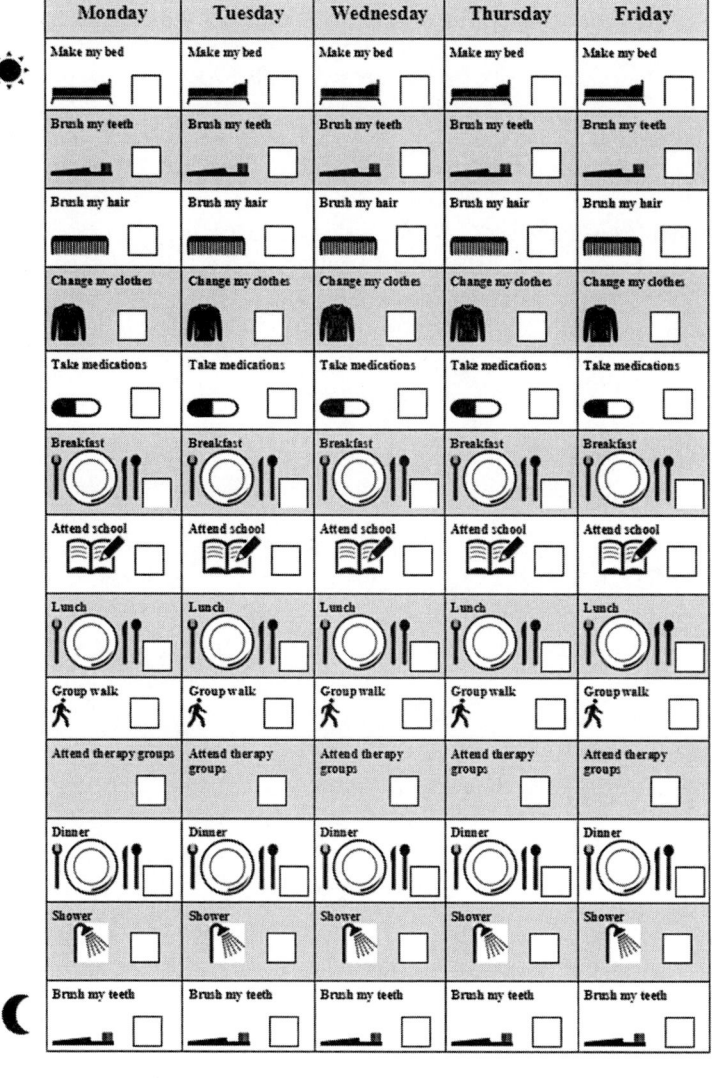

Fig. 13.2 Daily routine checklist

recipe, how she cleaned up afterwards), and transferred these findings to work with Bella in the other area of activities of daily living. A modified daily routine checklist was created for Bella to follow at home during her weekend leave. The occupational therapist met with Bella every Friday to plan and organise meaningful activity for her to do alone and with her family on the weekend (Fig. 13.3).

Children and adolescents with complex trauma or developmental impairments typically have difficulties with regulating their behaviours and emotions (Fraser et al., 2019) which can hinder their engagement in treatment. However, sensory-based interventions using sensorimotor experiences can help with self-regulating their affect to achieve optimal arousal for participating and engaging in treatment and daily life (Hitch et al., 2020). At the Walker Unit, sensory approaches are used extensively by the multidisciplinary team. In addition to supporting the young people in using sensory interventions, the occupational therapist at the Walker Unit

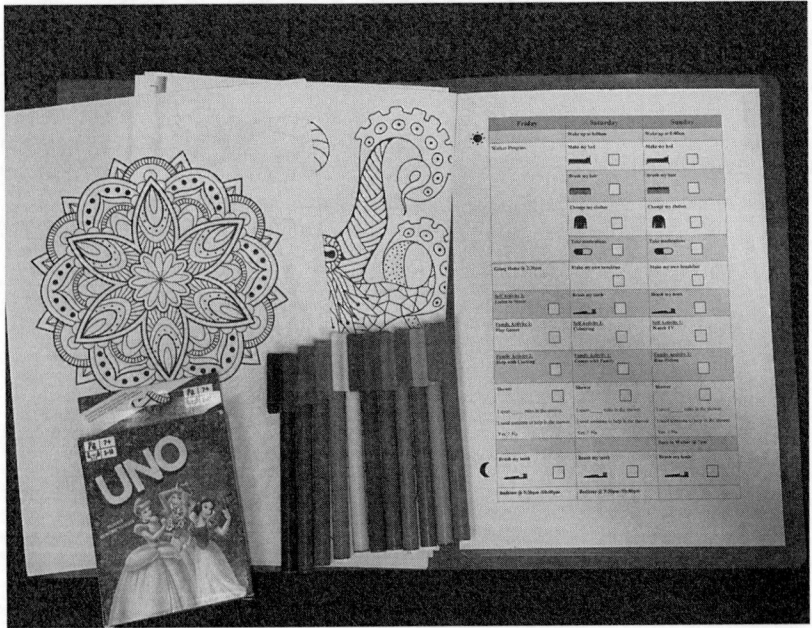

Fig. 13.3   Weekend activity pack including daily checklist and activities

also promotes and educates staff to integrate the sensory approaches into their therapeutic practice. After assessing the young person's sensory needs and in line with trauma-informed practice, the occupational therapist relies on the support from all members in the multidisciplinary team to support the use of the sensory interventions. For example, the occupational therapist will recommend the use of a weighted blanket and a rocking chair to help the individuals feel more bodily grounded and emotionally regulated or using intense stimulation like holding ice and strong scented room spray for orienting and distraction purposes. These interventions may be used by the multidisciplinary team in therapy settings (e.g. individual, group, family) and offered by nursing staff as de-escalation tools to encourage the young people to practice these strategies when they are distressed, and prevent restraint and seclusion use.

Sensory approaches are incorporated into the treatment environment of the Walker Unit. One of the interview rooms at the Walker Unit has been transformed into a sensory room (See Chap. 2). To overcome the lack of external windows a skylight was inserted in the ceiling. Features of the sensory room include a mural, massage chair, rocking chair, SenSit® chair, exercise balls, balance board, weighted blankets and a variety of fidgets and puzzles (Fig. 13.4). The sensory room provides not only a space for occupational therapy interventions; it has also been used as a therapy room for psychotherapy, group therapy or family therapy. Supervision is required when the young people are using the sensory room. Walker Unit also has a de-escalation room that provides a safe and low stimulus environment for the young people when needed. The Walker de-escalation room has a simple set up of a soft rocking chair, a lighting system with different colours and intensities and a sound system that connects with playlists selected by the music therapist. The de-escalation room can allow the young person to use this space unsupervised.

The Walker Unit team submitted a competitive funding proposal to transform the courtyards into two outdoor sensory gardens and was granted $40,000 for the project. With the support from the facility manager, the Walker Unit now has an uplifting, active garden and a calm, relaxing garden. The active garden promotes physical activities and has a trampoline, basketball hoop, table tennis table and exercise bike, all helping to uplift the energy of the young people (Fig. 13.5). The calm garden provides an outdoor space for the young people to chill out, with outdoor musical instruments like chimes and babel bells, sandpit, soft artificial

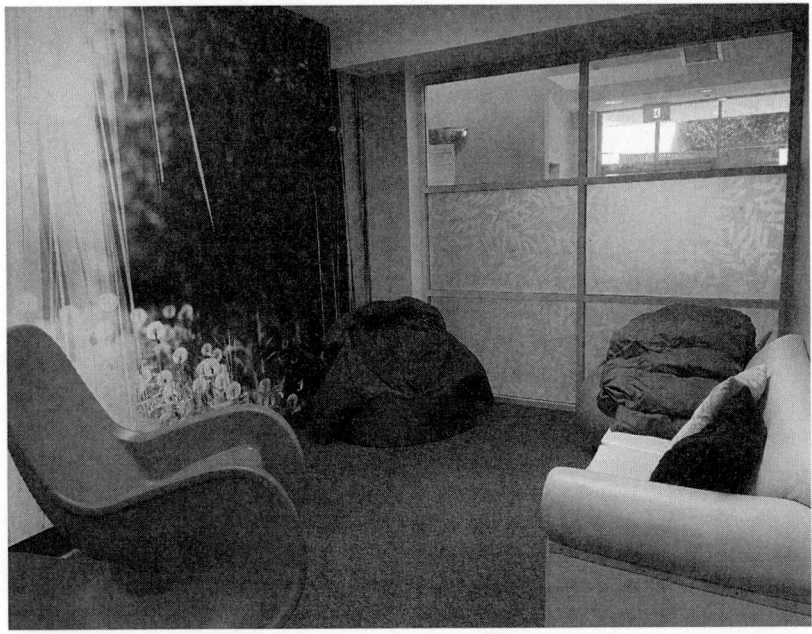

Fig. 13.4 The sensory room

lawn, water features, chalk painted wall, stepping stones, and planted with lavenders, edible herbs and fruit trees (Fig. 13.6).

With the thought of integrating the sensory approaches beyond the Walker Unit, personalised sensory kits are created with each young person (Champagne, 2011). The young person decides the purpose of the personalised sensory kits and organises the most helpful items according to their specific needs. This way, the sensory kit would be readily available to the young person when they are distressed. Furthermore, all clinicians from the multidisciplinary team can support the young people using the sensory kit. A sensory kit may include fidget toys, stress balls, scented hand lotion, strong mints, sour lollies, journal and a colouring in or puzzle book. The young people are encouraged to take their personalised sensory kits to therapy sessions, school or home. The personalised sensory kits are safe interventions to use in this restrictive environment in terms of infection control and risk of harm (Fig. 13.7).

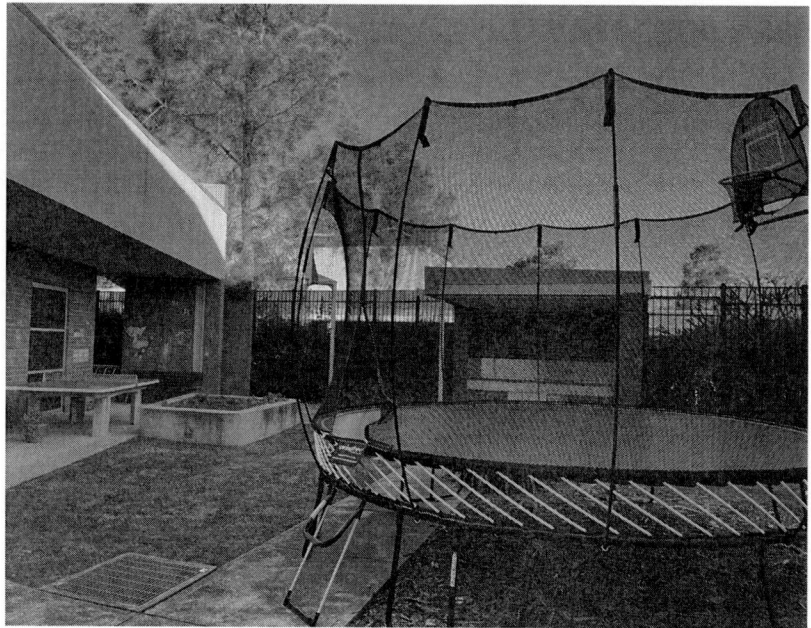

Fig. 13.5 The active garden

The following case example illustrates the sensory approach directed to a young person:

Carl was a 16 years old boy who enjoyed poetry and skateboarding. He always wore the same sport jacket and track pants even in warm weather. He was isolative, disorganised, neglected self-care, and had difficulties with social relationships and communication. Carl experienced persecutory delusions, and engaged in bizarre behaviours. He was irritable and could at times be threatening. In the face of limit-setting he would become distressed, agitated and aggressive. He had a history of oppositional and rule-breaking behaviour, but he had responded well to the behaviour management plan. He continued to struggle to participate in the group program and verbal therapy. The occupational therapist engaged Carl in non-verbal therapy utilising sensory approaches. The therapy sessions included walks around the hospital grounds listening to his favourite rap music, in order for Carl to

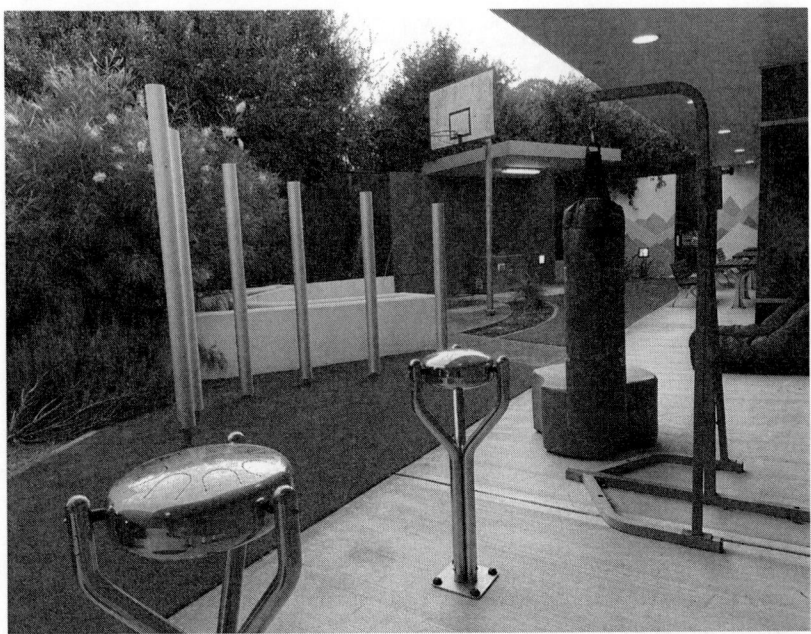

Fig. 13.6 The calm garden

practice his skateboarding skills as well as having sensory input to regulate his behaviours; as a grounding strategy the occupational therapist also used sand play and chalk art for Carl to express himself and swimming in the hospital pool to help Carl to "clear his thoughts".

Conclusion

The occupational therapist at the Walker Unit uses creative ways to engage the young people achieving their goals and enhancing their functions. The occupational therapist work closely with the multidisciplinary team, support from the Walker team is crucial for all occupational therapy interventions.

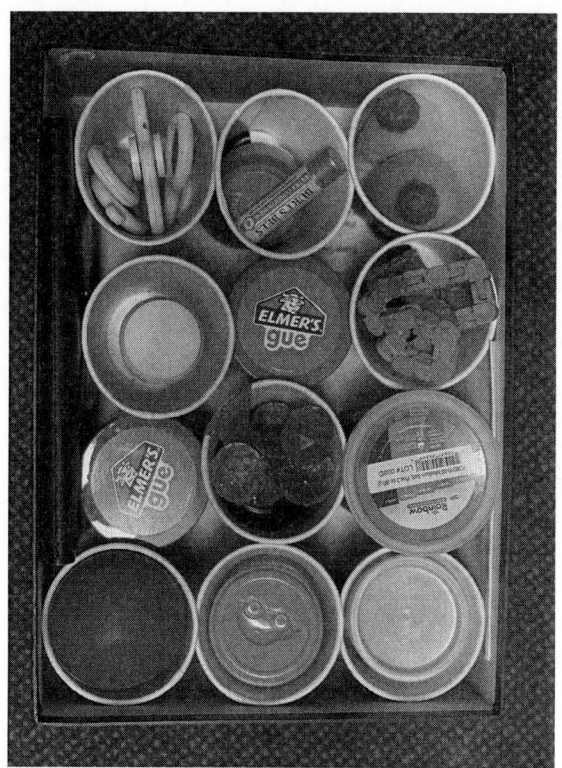

Fig. 13.7 Personalised sensory box

REFERENCES

Champagne, T. (2011). *Sensory modulation and environment: Essential elements of occupation* (3rd ed.). Pearson.

Fossey, E., & Bramley, S. (2014). Work and vocational pursuits. In J. F. W. Bryan & K. Bannigan (Eds.), *Creek's occupational therapy and mental health* (pp. 328–344). Churchill Livingstone.

Fraser, K., MacKenzie, D., & Versnel, J. (2019). What is the current state of occupational therapy practice with children and adolescents with complex trauma? *Occupational Therapy in Mental Health, 35*(4), 317–338. https://doi.org/10.1080/0164212X.2019.1652132

Hitch, D., Wilson, C., & A., H. (2020). Sensory modulation in mental health practice. *Mental Health Practice, 23*(3), 11–16. https://doi.org/10.7748/mhp.2020.e1422

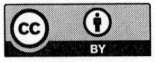

CHAPTER 14

Speech and Language Therapy

Kelly Jones

Abstract There is a multi-directional relationship between communication difficulties and mental health. A young person with a language disorder may fall behind at school, have difficulty maintaining appropriate peer relationships and have trouble expressing their internal experience. This can result in adverse mental health outcomes. Conversely, a mental health condition which leads to a young person not attending school and withdrawing from family and friends alters the environmental input they receive in terms of speech, language and social communication; they may therefore fall behind in these areas. It is also important to recognise that communication impairments are inherent in a number of mental health conditions—for example, marked changes to speech rate and language content in psychoses.

Keywords Adolescent • Inpatients • Mental health • Speech-language pathology • Communication disorders

K. Jones (✉)
Concord Centre for Mental Health, Concord, NSW, Australia
e-mail: Kelly.Jones1@health.nsw.gov.au

© The Author(s) 2022   127
P. Hazell (ed.), *Longer-Term Psychiatric Inpatient Care for Adolescents*, https://doi.org/10.1007/978-981-19-1950-3_14

INTRODUCTION

A senior speech pathologist is a member of the multidisciplinary team (MDT) at the Walker Unit. The speech pathologist assesses the communication needs of the young people and diagnoses any potential communication impairments. They also collaborate with the MDT to modify the ward programme and materials, such as care plans, to ensure they are accessible for varying levels of communication ability. The speech pathologist acts as a consultant to the unit on communication matters, while also providing direct interventions to young people either individually or in groups.

The Walker Unit recognises the importance of determining any underlying communication difficulties and tailoring its service to the communication needs of an individual young person. This chapter will explore the work of speech pathologists on the unit. It should be noted that speech pathologists also assess and manage dysphagia (swallowing difficulties). Management of dysphagia is not a common requirement at the Walker Unit however and thus this chapter will focus on communication.

SIGNS OF COMMUNICATION DIFFICULTY

Effective communication is the expression of wants, needs and feelings by the "sender" or "speaker" and the accurate interpretation or comprehension of these by a "receiver" or "listener". Communication is not simply talking; other communication skills include hearing, listening, understanding, social skills, reading and writing (Speech Pathology Australia, 2010). Non-verbal communication is just as valid a means of communication as speaking and at times is easier for people to engage with.

When working with a young person the following may be signs of communication difficulty:

- misinterpreting questions or instructions (i.e. giving "strange" or unrelated answers, doing a task differently than how they were told or not at all)
- limited vocabulary when explaining their thoughts, opinions and feelings,
- difficulty with school work or reluctance to attend school
- requiring additional time to complete tasks

- appearing to be behind in conversation, that is, seeming not to recognise when the topic has moved on
- difficulty interpreting sarcasm, understanding jokes and reading the body language of others
- not initiating any interactions and/or when asked questions giving one or two word responses

Why it Is Important to Recognise Communication Difficulties

Communication difficulties during childhood and adolescence can significantly impact on an individual's psychosocial outcomes, educational attainment and wider social experience. Research has shown the links between communication abilities and education outcomes (Conti-Ramsden et al., 2009), self-esteem (Jerome et al., 2002), peer relationships (Durkin & Conti-Ramsden, 2007) and externalising behaviours (James et al., 2020; Maggio et al., 2014).

Those with a communication disorder in early life are at greater risk of particular mental health conditions (Arkkila et al., 2008; Charman et al., 2015). Furthermore, communication difficulties have implications for a young person's ability to engage in mental health treatment (Conti-Ramsden et al., 2013).

Speech Pathology at the Walker Unit

At the Walker unit, the speech pathologist is part of the "in-house" team rather than an ad hoc referral service. This is an important point of difference compared to many other mental health services. When a speech pathologist is included in the team, they have greater opportunity to identify and support the communication needs of the young people. As such, the speech pathologist participates in all patient care meetings, ranging from daily handover to bi-monthly mini-team meetings. Due to the at times volatile or changeable nature of complex mental health admissions communication supports may be needed with little notice and having the speech pathologist onsite allows for a prompt intervention.

When a young person is admitted to the Walker Unit the speech pathologist screens their history to identify any information which could signify the need for communication supports, including but not limited to a consideration of mental health diagnosis, a prior diagnosis of a communication disorder, hearing ability, literacy, academic performance, and conditions that frequently present with communication differences or difficulties such as autism spectrum disorder (ASD), attention deficit hyperactivity disorder (ADHD), and intellectual disability.

Formal communication assessment may be required as part of the diagnostic work up. Formal and informal communication assessment will also occur if the speech pathologist identifies behaviours which could indicate previously undiagnosed difficulties. Assessment and intervention may need to be adapted for young people of culturally and linguistically diverse backgrounds. Examples of adaption include the use of interpreters, the exclusion of particular assessments which rely on background cultural knowledge or idioms, and/or the use of subtests from some standardised assessments used instead informally as sources of qualitative information rather than to get standard scores.

Formal assessment, where a young person can be compared to aged matched peers, may include the Clinical Evaluation of Language Fundamentals (Wiig & Secord, 2014; Wiig et al., 2013), the Test for Reception of Grammar (Bishop, 2003), the Peabody Picture Vocabulary test (Dunn, 2019), the Expressive Vocabulary test (Williams, 2019), and/or The Awareness of Social Inference Test—Revised (McDonald et al., 2011), and Social Language Development Test (Bowers et al., 2017), depending on the clinical question. None of the instruments listed were designed specifically for use with young people in a mental health setting. As such, speech pathologists must use their best clinical judgement to determine the most appropriate instrument for each young person.

Informal assessment refers to non-standardised non-normed observations and information collection. This can occur in a variety of ways and may gather information from a range of communication partners including family, teachers, nursing and other clinical staff. Methods can include semi structured interviews, pragmatic profiles (see e.g. Dewart & Summers, 1996), communication checklists, and observations made by the speech pathologist of the young person in different group settings, during different activities on the ward and with different people. Young people are always asked about their own view of their communication, including strengths and challenges. This includes who the young person finds it easy or easiest to communicate with and in what contexts. Self-report may be facilitated by the use of checklists such as those in the Talkabout manuals (Kelly & Bains, 2017; Kelly et al., 2019). Additionally, insight and motivation are important to ascertain at assessment to determine approach to intervention (i.e. direct or environmental). A long period of rapport building is often necessary to gain the trust of the young person, so that they will engage in these interactions.

At the Walker Unit, in addition to a comprehensive assessment report, a simple language version is created and shared with the carer and/or young person. This supports comprehension of the assessment results bearing in mind that families may also have communication difficulties (Kang & Drayna, 2011). Additionally, reports for disability support funding agencies (in Australia, the National Disability Insurance Scheme) may provide further support for access to the scheme and/or result in funding for the young person to continue receiving particular supports post discharge which may include seeing a speech pathologist.

The target for any direct intervention is determined in collaboration with the young person, working with their motivation. For example, a young person with a severe language disorder and social communication difficulties identified the most important thing for them was not being the "stupid" one in their grade. When this was explored further they were able to identify that they felt "stupid" when they did not understand what other people were laughing or joking about. The focus was therefore on vocabulary, in particular multi-meaning words and inferencing. This contributed to them feeling more comfortable around their peers and supported their wider receptive language skills.

The speech pathologist works collaboratively with the art and music therapists to support non-verbal expression and when appropriate, supports the young person to put words to their experience. At times, the speech pathologist may work with the young person to create or document their emotional "vocabulary". This does not necessarily mean changing the words the young person uses for their experience. More often it will take the form of documenting what these words actually mean or signal for the young person so that those caring for them can understand what they are trying to communicate. For example, one young person may use the word "ok" to describe a sense of calm whilst for someone else this may mean "I'm feeling on the verge of self-harm".

The speech pathologist often uses visual aids to support communication. Comic Strip Conversations (Gray, 1994) is an example of a visual approach that the speech pathologist may use with young people at the Walker Unit. The approach uses drawings and colours to visually represent different perspectives in social situations. Individuals can benefit from this as it makes the more abstract aspects of social communication easier to understand. The approach can be used to explore social difficulties that occur, considering what is said as well as thoughts and feelings (which are visually represented). It can also be used to consider different outcomes that could result from different ways of interacting (see Figs. 14.1a and 14.1b). Another visual aid is Talking Mats ™ (Murphy & Cameron, 2006), an interactive resource that can be used to support comprehension, and to facilitate expression of feelings and opinions. It uses sets of cards which show a picture and word relating to various topics. This resource can reduce the cognitive load required for communication and facilitate expression for those who find it difficult to verbalise, whether this be due to anxiety or a communication disorder. Furthermore, it does not require literacy skills which is beneficial, given well established links between literacy difficulties and emotional and behavioural conditions (Hurry et al., 2018).

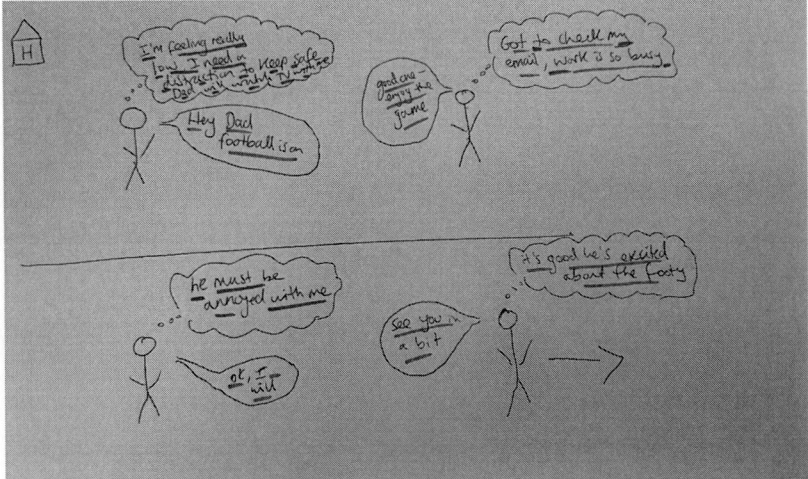

Fig. 14.1a Comic Strip Conversation, using the methodology of Carol Gray (1994) exploring an interaction with a young person and their Father. What was said is shown in speech bubbles, what was thought by the young person and potentially thought by the father is shown in thought bubbles and the way these things were said/potential feelings is shown by the colours. In this case green represents a friendly or relaxed feeling and blue represents an uncomfortable or stressed feeling

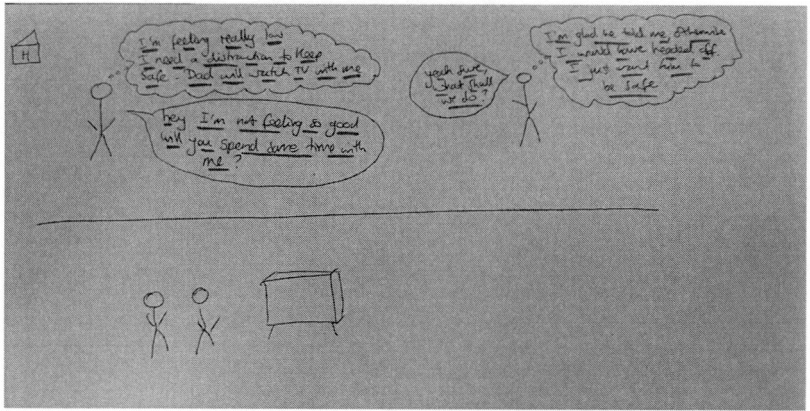

Fig. 14.1b Following on from the event in Fig. 14.1a this image depicts what could have happened if the young person had said something different in the same situation

A diagnosis of a communication disorder or determination of particular communication needs can be new information for carers. Education on these topics can raise awareness and change behaviour in terms of interactions amongst family members. When needed, the speech pathologist works with carers to consider different communication profiles, provide communication partner education and/or training to facilitate more effective or enjoyable interactions.

A number of communication groups have been run by speech pathologists at the Walker Unit, which have targeted basic communication skills such as having an awareness of self and others, through to groups which focus on more complex pragmatic skills such as how to start and keep conversations going. Talkabout resources (Kelly & Bains, 2017; Kelly et al., 2019) are an example of resources used to support group content. In other circumstances, the speech pathologist contributes by advising how a ward group may need to adapt to the specific communication needs of young people.

CONCLUSION

A large number of young people with mental health conditions have communication difficulties. Staff at the Walker Unit have the skills and indeed a responsibility to use communication that is accessible to an adolescent cohort. The specific skills of the speech pathologist are required when a young person has additional communication needs.

REFERENCES

Arkkila, E., Rasanen, P., Roine, R. P., & Vilkman, E. (2008). Specific language impairment in childhood is associated with impaired mental and social well-being in adulthood. *Logopedics, Phoniatrics, Vocology, 33*(4), 179–189. https://doi.org/10.1080/14015430802088289

Bishop, D. V. M. (2003). *Test of reception of grammar version 2 (TROG-2.).* Pearson Assessment.

Bowers, L., Huisingh, R., & Lo Giudice, C. (2017). *Social language development test—Adolescent: normative update.* Pro-ed.

Charman, T., Ricketts, J., Dockrell, J. E., Lindsay, G., & Palikara, O. (2015). Emotional and behavioural problems in children with language impairments and children with autism spectrum disorders. *International Journal of Language & Communication Disorders, 50*(1), 84–93. https://doi.org/10.1111/1460-6984.12116

Conti-Ramsden, G., Durkin, K., Simkin, Z., & Knox, E. (2009). Specific language impairment and school outcomes. I: Identifying and explaining variability at the end of compulsory education. *International Journal of Language & Communication Disorders, 44*(1), 15–35. https://doi.org/10.1080/13682820801921601

Conti-Ramsden, G., Mok, P. L., Pickles, A., & Durkin, K. (2013). Adolescents with a history of specific language impairment (SLI): Strengths and difficulties in social, emotional and behavioral functioning. *Research in Developmental Disabilities, 34*(11), 4161–4169. https://doi.org/10.1016/j.ridd.2013.08.043

Dewart, H., & Summers, S. T. (1996). *The pragmatics profile of everyday communication skills in adults.* NFER-NELSON.

Dunn, D. M. (2019). *Peabody picture vocabulary test* (5th ed.). NCS Pearson.

Durkin, K., & Conti-Ramsden, G. (2007). Language, social behavior, and the quality of friendships in adolescents with and without a history of specific language impairment. *Child Development, 78*(5), 1441–1457. https://doi.org/10.1111/j.1467-8624.2007.01076.x

Gray, C. (1994). *Comic strip conversations: Illustrated interactions that teach conversation skills to students with autism and related disorders.* Future Horizons.

Hurry, J., Flouri, E., & Sylva, K. (2018). Literacy difficulties and emotional and behavior disorders: Causes and consequences. *Journal of Education for Students Placed at Risk, 23*(3), 259–279. https://doi.org/10.1080/1082466 9.2018.1482748

James, K., Munro, N., Togher, L., & Cordier, R. (2020). The spoken language and social communication characteristics of adolescents in Behavioral schools: A controlled comparison study. *Language, Speech, and Hearing Services in Schools, 51*(1), 115–127. https://doi.org/10.1044/2019_lshss-18-0090

Jerome, A. C., Fujiki, M., Brinton, B., & James, S. L. (2002). Self-esteem in children with specific language impairment. *Journal of Speech, Language, and Hearing Research, 45*(4), 700–714. https://doi.org/10.1044/ 1092-4388(2002/056)

Kang, C., & Drayna, D. (2011). Genetics of speech and language disorders. *Annual Review of Genomics and Human Genetics, 12*, 145–164. https://doi. org/10.1146/annurev-genom-090810-183119

Kelly, A., & Bains, S. (2017). *Talkabout for teenagers: Developing social and emotional communication skills* (2nd ed.). Taylor & Francis Ltd..

Kelly, A., Tarshis, N., & Meringolo, D. (2019). *Talkabout: A social communication skills package.* Routledge.

Maggio, V., Grañana, N. E., Richaudeau, A., Torres, S., Giannotti, A., & Suburo, A. M. (2014). Behavior problems in children with specific language impairment. *Journal of Child Neurology, 29*(2), 194–202. https://doi. org/10.1177/0883073813509886

McDonald, S., Flanagan, S., & Rollins, J. (2011). *The awareness of social inference test (revised).* Pearson Assessment.

Murphy, J., & Cameron, L. (2006). *Talking Mats: A resource to enhance communication.* University of Stirling.

Speech Pathology Australia. (2010). *Speech pathology in mental health services clinical guideline.* Retrieved 28 Sept, 2021, from www.speechpathologyaustralia.org.au/SPAweb/Members/Clinical_Guidelines/spaweb/Members/ Clinical_Guidelines/Clinical_Guidelines.aspx?hkey=f66634e4-825a-4f1a-910d-644553f59140

Wiig, E. H., & Secord, W. A. (2014). *Clinical evaluation of language fundamentals, fifth edition metalinguistics (CELF®-5 metalinguistics).* NCS Pearson.

Wiig, E. H., Semel, E., & Secord, W. A. (2013). *Clinical evaluation of language fundamentals –fifth edition.* NCS Pearson.

Williams, K. T. (2019). *Expressive vocabulary test* (3rd ed.). NCS Pearson.

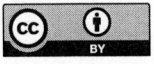

CHAPTER 15

Food and Eating

Kia Currell and Polly Kwan

Abstract The Walker Unit recognises the role of good nutrition to help support a young person's growth and mental health. An experienced dietician and chef work closely with patients, families and staff to ensure dietary needs and meal preferences are managed to support good mental and physical health. The multidisciplinary team at the Walker Unit have experience managing difficult and complex eating behaviours that can present along with severe mental illness. These include restrictive and avoidant eating behaviours, overeating and binge eating, compensatory behaviours following eating, poor eating routines, increased appetite and cardiometabolic side effects of some treatments. The Walker Unit team recognise that these complex eating behaviours may require management from different and often creative angles which require the skillset of a multidisciplinary team.

Keywords Adolescent • Inpatients • Mental Health • Diet, Healthy • Nutrition Policy

K. Currell • P. Kwan (✉)
Walker Unit, Concord Centre for Mental Health, Concord, NSW, Australia
e-mail: Kia.Currell@health.nsw.gov.au; Polly.Kwan@health.nsw.gov.au

© The Author(s) 2022   137
P. Hazell (ed.), *Longer-Term Psychiatric Inpatient Care for Adolescents*, https://doi.org/10.1007/978-981-19-1950-3_15

INTRODUCTION

The role of nutrition supporting mental health is a growing field of research. Across mental health populations nutrition concerns may manifest as a side effects of antipsychotic medications (e.g. weight gain and poor cardiometabolic health), disordered eating behaviours (e.g. food restriction, binge eating) or general poor diet quality contributing to mental health symptoms (Barton et al., 2020; Bretler et al., 2019; Firth et al., 2019; Jacka et al., 2017). The Walker Unit must address these concerns while at the same time maintaining adequate nutrition to support normal adolescent growth and development.

COMPLEX EATING BEHAVIOURS

A key issue for staff at the Walker Unit is managing the balance between vastly different nutrition concerns and presentations. For example managing meal times and nutrition plans for consumers who are under nourished and those who are over nourished. Consumers who are undernourished may be required to have additional and more desirable snacks and meals than those who are over nourished and aiming to limit these food options for overall health improvements. While individually these management plans are straightforward, in the group dining room setting at meal times, this can lead to challenging behaviour for nursing staff to manage. For example, other consumers may see a lack of equality between food provided to them versus other consumers. Successful techniques staff have found to help manage this include having strong consistent messages amongst staff supervising meals, reinforcing that all consumer have different goals and plans, use of high energy nutritional supplement drinks for consumers experiencing under nutrition to add to the diet rather than copious amounts of discretionary foods which may trigger dietary comparisons amongst patients.

As consumers progress through the Walker programme, and increased time is spent at home and or school, the young person's nutrition plan must be adapted to suit the change in environment. At this point, the routine and control of the Walker meal structure is altered. Sometimes there is a recurrence of previous abnormal eating, for example binge eating in the context of uncontrolled food availability. At this stage, it is important to liaise with the family network to ensure meal times and portions are kept consistent with the Walker programme to help ensure an easier transition. This is also a prime opportunity for introducing new foods and food environments which may present challenges. During this transition, it is common for eating habits to regress slightly as the consumer manages the many emotions and challenges experienced with the transition.

CREATIVE ANGLES FOR NUTRITION MANAGEMENT

Early in the evolution of the Walker programme a position of 'Living Skills Cook' was created to enable young people to receive freshly cooked meals tailored to their needs. A chef with excellent people skills is employed on weekdays to prepare morning tea, lunch, afternoon tea and dinner. Nursing staff provide breakfast and supper. This model aims to replicate home-style cooking which young people are familiar with and helps to reduce the feeling of institutionalisation (Hartwell et al., 2013). Young people attend meals in a communal dining area and eat with staff. This model allows for choice of meals at the point of service which has been shown to enhance consumer meal satisfaction and in turn assist with achieving nutritional adequacy (Mahoney et al., 2009). On weekends, the unit's meals are supplied by the hospital's centralised kitchen. Monotony is relieved by a Saturday breakfast group, run by the occupational therapist, the opportunity for food to be sent in by families, and occasional take-away meals.

The chef receives guidance from the Food Service dietician to ensure meals prepared meet the nutritional requirements for adolescents and are appropriate for this group. This is of particular importance given most young people at the Walker Unit have longer admissions and are predominantly reliant on the hospital provided meals to meet their nutritional requirements. The chef liaises with the staff and young people to ensure the menu is tailored to meet their needs and preferences. The dietician also works closely with the chef to ensure young people with special nutritional needs are well managed. For example, young people requiring a meal plan will have this meal plan organised with the chef to ensure appropriate meal variety and options are available.

The nutrition guide for the Walker Unit aims to provide adequate variety and quantity of all core food groups for adolescents as per the Australian Guide to Healthy Eating for Children and teenagers (Australian Government Department of Health, 2015). Of particular focus for the Walker Unit is vegetarian diets. Often vegetarian diets are requested for ethical and cultural reasons, though at times, they are requested by consumers aiming to restrict their caloric intake. The nutrition guideline developed for the Walker Unit ensures that the protein requirements and iron requirements are met for those requesting vegetarian meals, which often requires education and up skilling with the chef. The chef is then able to creatively implement this to help reduce menu fatigue.

Cooking interventions have been frequently used by occupational therapists in a wide range of clinical settings, with the aims to provide consumers with opportunities for developing life skills, their identity and social relationships among the peers (Farmer et al., 2018). Some young people admitted to the unit have never cooked a meal. Others, owing to circumstances, have had limited opportunity to learn how to cook (Utter et al., 2016).

Cooking groups are used at the Walker Unit to provide the young people with cooking experiences. Each week, the young people would be supported to have a group discussion and make a choice of the recipes for the cooking groups. This provides an opportunity for the young people to try new food or select a culture specific cuisine. Young people are also encouraged to bring in recipes from home for the cooking groups. Young people will be supported to work together during the cooking task, practice social and negotiation skills, learn how to prepare simple meals from basic ingredients. Cooking interventions improve eating behaviour, self-esteem, confidence, concentration, coordination, and provide a sense of achievement (Farmer et al., 2018) (Fig. 15.1).

While diet quality is an important consideration for consumers at the Walker Unit, promoting and demonstrating a healthy meal environment is of equal importance. Young people often have not had a positive meal environment for some time prior to their admission to the Walker Unit, and are unaware what constitutes acceptable and normal mealtime behaviour. At the Walker Unit, young people consume all meals in a central dining room area which helps create a family meal sharing experience. Staff also sit at the dining table and consume the same meal provided, again, to encourage a normalised meal experience. During this time, distractions such as phones and television are restricted. The practice of communal meals has also been shown to have positive nutritional outcomes including improved motivation to consume meals, increased meal satisfaction as well as non-nutritional improvements including enhanced socialisation skills (Hartwell et al., 2013).

Staff from all disciplines eat meals with the young people. Doing so affords the opportunity to model normal eating behaviours such as consuming appropriate quantities, embracing a variety of foods, and engaging in socially appropriate conversations while dining. It also affords the opportunity for staff to provide meal support for consumers when needed.

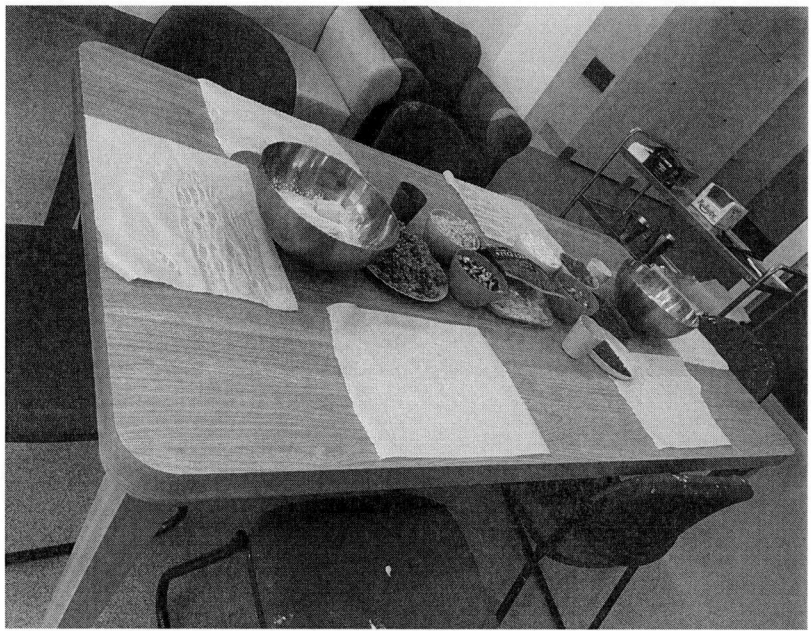

Fig. 15.1 Example cooking group set up

For example, young people who are struggling to eat may require regular prompting to consume an adequate amount. Nursing staff also keep food charts and records for consumers if the dietician requests, to help identify meal patterns and if dietary intake is adequate. Finally, sharing a meal is an excellent way for staff to build rapport with the young people.

Overeating and undereating are common challenges. This was previously managed with individualised meal plans for each young person to help them consume an adequate intake. After consultation with the ward chef, this process was found to be confusing for staff around adequate portions to be served at main meals. To help address this the ward chef and dietician developed three pictorial meal plans utilising food and utensils commonly used on the ward to demonstrate consistent portions for young people who need to increase or decrease their intake. See example below (Fig. 15.2).

The following case example illustrates a collaborative, non-coercive approach to the management of undereating:

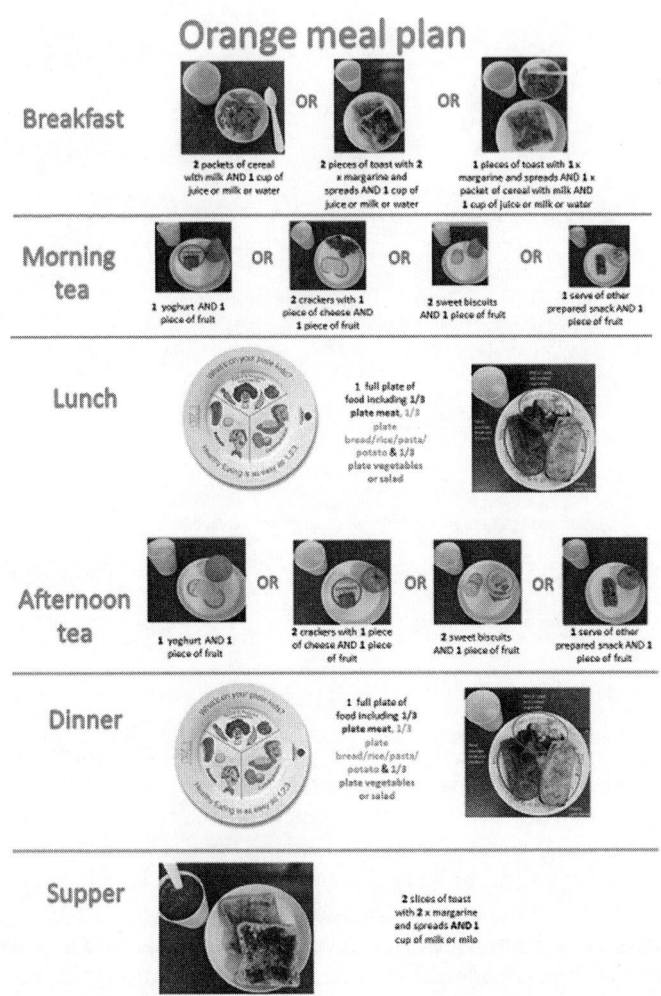

Fig. 15.2 Example pictorial meal guide for Walker consumers

A 16 year old female transitioning to male was referred to the Walker Unit dietician on admission with a request for a vegan diet. The young person had a low body weight, minimal dietary intake, and was severely malnourished. Amongst other concerns there was a risk for refeeding syndrome. The young person was not agreeable, at this stage, to any food offered and was refusing engagement with most aspects of the ward programme. Initial interventions were focused on managing the young person's risk of refeeding syndrome and increasing their dietary intake. As rapport was established with selected team members, the young person became more agreeable to engaging in dietary interventions. This included initially consuming familiar food provided by family, and familiar hospital food consumed during a previous hospitalisation. Nursing staff maintained food and weight charts. Staff consistently offered and encouraged dietary intake at regular meal times to help encourage the young person increase their intake. In addition to this the young person was prescribed high energy high protein nutritional supplementation to further increase their nutritional intake. After several weeks of this consistent approach the young person started to initiate consumption of meals independently and increased their dietary intake at all meals. The young person became more amenable to trying unfamiliar meals prepared by the ward chef. The young person met with the ward chef and a nursing staff member to discuss meal preferences which further helped to enhance engagement in dietary intake. The young person experienced body image concerns related to their mental health and gender dysphoria which had an impact on their eating habits throughout the earlier part of their admission and coincided with some relapses in dietary intake. With consistent support from staff and open communication with the family and consumer with regards to appropriate food from home, the young person was able to establish a healthy dietary intake. As the consumer became more settled into the ward they started actively engaging in regular cooking groups and individual cooking sessions with the occupational therapist. This included baking a birthday cake for a family member for weekend leave. Prior to leaving the Walker Unit the young person was able to achieve and maintain a healthy weight with dietary intake alone (no nutritional supplementation).

References

Australian Government Department of Health. (2015). Eat for health. Healthy eating for children. Retrieved September 2, 2021, from https://www.eatforhealth.gov.au/sites/default/files/content/The%20Guidelines/n55f_children_brochure.pdf

Barton, B. B., Segger, F., Fischer, K., Obermeier, M., & Musil, R. (2020). Update on weight-gain caused by antipsychotics: A systematic review and meta-analysis. *Expert Opinion on Drug Safety, 19*(3), 295–314. https://doi.org/10.1080/14740338.2020.1713091

Bretler, T., Weisberg, H., Koren, O., & Neuman, H. (2019). The effects of antipsychotic medications on microbiome and weight gain in children and adolescents. *BMC Medicine, 17*(1), 112. https://doi.org/10.1186/s12916-019-1346-1

Farmer, N., Touchton-Leonard, K., & Ross, A. (2018). Psychosocial benefits of cooking interventions: A systematic review. *Health Education & Behavior, 45*(2), 167–180. https://doi.org/10.1177/1090198117736352

Firth, J., Siddiqi, N., Koyanagi, A., Siskind, D., Rosenbaum, S., Galletly, C., Allan, S., Caneo, C., Carney, R., Carvalho, A. F., Chatterton, M. L., Correll, C. U., Curtis, J., Gaughran, F., Heald, A., Hoare, E., Jackson, S. E., Kisely, S., Lovell, K., … Stubbs, B. (2019). The Lancet Psychiatry Commission: A blueprint for protecting physical health in people with mental illness. *Lancet Psychiatry, 6*(8), 675–712. https://doi.org/10.1016/s2215-0366(19)30132-4

Hartwell, H. J., Shepherd, P. A., & Edwards, J. S. A. (2013). Effects of a hospital ward eating environment on patients' mealtime experience: A pilot study. *Nutrition & Dietetics, 70*(4), 332–338. https://doi.org/10.1111/1747-0080.12042

Jacka, F. N., O'Neil, A., Opie, R., Itsiopoulos, C., Cotton, S., Mohebbi, M., Castle, D., Dash, S., Mihalopoulos, C., Chatterton, M. L., Brazionis, L., Dean, O. M., Hodge, A. M., & Berk, M. (2017). A randomised controlled trial of dietary improvement for adults with major depression (the 'SMILES' trial). *BMC Medicine, 15*(1), 23. https://doi.org/10.1186/s12916-017-0791-y

Mahoney, S., Zulli, A., & Walton, K. (2009). Patient satisfaction and energy intakes are enhanced by point of service meal provision. *Nutrition & Dietetics, 66*(4), 212–220. https://doi.org/10.1111/j.1747-0080.2009.01373.x

Utter, J., Denny, S., Lucassen, M., & Dyson, B. (2016). Adolescent cooking abilities and behaviors: Associations with nutrition and emotional well-being. *Journal of Nutrition Education and Behavior, 48*(1), 35–41.e31. https://doi.org/10.1016/j.jneb.2015.08.016

CHAPTER 16

Physical Wellbeing

Ariel Diaz and Philip Hazell

Abstract Regular physical exertion is protective against depression, promotes healthy sleep and may counteract the adverse metabolic effects of psychotropic agents. The Walker programme benefited for a time from the input of a sports psychologist, who provided tailored exercise programmes for most patients. The nursing team has continued to champion physical activity through use of an exercycle and rowing machine, 'beep' tests, group walks and games. Seizure disorders and Type 1 diabetes are the most common comorbid medical problems amongst the patient population, and usually require physician consultation. Metabolic health is monitored and managed per protocol when patients are prescribed second generation antipsychotics. Surgical problems arising from self-harm are common and include laceration, wound interference, ingestion of objects, and insertion of objects.

A. Diaz
Walker Unit, Concord Centre for Mental Health, Concord, NSW, Australia
e-mail: Ariel.Diaz@health.nsw.gov.au

P. Hazell (✉)
Walker Unit, Concord Centre for Mental Health, Concord, NSW, Australia

The University of Sydney, Sydney, NSW, Australia
e-mail: Philip.Hazell@health.nsw.gov.au

© The Author(s) 2022
P. Hazell (ed.), *Longer-Term Psychiatric Inpatient Care for Adolescents*, https://doi.org/10.1007/978-981-19-1950-3_16

Keywords Adolescent • Inpatients • Mental Health • Overweight • Exercise Therapy

Metabolic Wellbeing

Mental illness, especially that impairing enough to warrant hospitalisation in a longer stay high severity unit, is associated with poor physical health. Lifestyle factors typical of the experience of mental illness such as poor diet, poor sleep, substance misuse and lack of physical activity contribute to overweight and its associated health problems (Carney, 2019). The metabolic effects of psychotropic medications commonly prescribed in the inpatient setting add to the risk. Psychiatric inpatient units for adolescents have been described as 'obesogenic' (Carney, 2019). Characteristics of the mental health ward environment thought to contribute to obesity include (Carney, 2019):

- Fewer opportunities to be physically active
- Increased time spent engaged in sedentary activity
- Restricted living space and general daily activity
- Increased severity of symptoms such as low mood, anxiety and symptoms of psychosis
- Increased access to highly calorific and nutritionally poor foods
- Low access to home-cooked foods due to restrictions on foods allowed on the wards
- Side-effects of medication (e.g. those prescribed antipsychotics)
- 'Culture' of the inpatient wards, for example, pizza night

Strategies to improve the situation include attention to nutrition, increased physical activity, and systematic monitoring (Carney, 2019). The nutritional interventions employed at the Walker Unit are described in Chap. 15, while the monitoring of patients prescribed medications known to have metabolic effects is described in Chap. 17. Features of the ward environment that promote physical activity are summarised in Chap. 2. A systematic review of interventions to improve physical health among adolescents on mental health inpatient units identified no studies that focussed on nutrition (Carney et al., 2021). Two uncontrolled 'before and after' design studies of enhanced physical activity were identified. In one study, there was an aggregate improvement in Health of the Nation Outcome Scale for Children and Adolescents scores, while in another there was an aggregate reduction in Body Mass Index (BMI) and waist circumference, and a concurrent lowering of resting pulse rate. The review identified one uncontrolled study of yoga which found an improvement in behaviour rating scale scores and a reduction in the number of behavioural interventions required (Carney et al., 2021). Given the high prevalence of physical health problems among adolescent psychiatric inpatients (Eapen et al., 2012) the lack of empirical research examining intervention is concerning.

During its short history, the Walker Unit has at times had access to the expertise of a sports psychologist and an exercise physiologist. Funding constraints have meant that neither position could be sustained long-term. Activities initiated by the psychologist and physiologist have, however, been continued by the nursing staff. One such activity is the sports group. It was introduced as a fun activity that to promote physical health in conjunction with mental health. Many studies show that physical health improves mental health, especially with regards to depression. The group is run twice a week for one hour each of those days. Both indoor and outdoor activities are available, with the use of the courtyard and large lounge areas of the ward being utilised for days when patients are unable to go out to the adjacent Rivendell grounds due to either safety or poor weather. During the weekly community meeting, patients are encouraged to come up with suggestions as to what physical activity they would prefer to do that given week—usually choosing an outdoor and indoor activity. Some activities include basketball, dodge ball, swimming (utilising hospital communal pool), jumping on the ward trampoline, soccer, tennis, ping-pong amongst other creative games invented by the nursing staff—especially in the limited indoor environment. There is a combined sports group run once per week with an adjacent adolescent inpatient unit and day hospital catering for young people with moderately severe mental illness. The combined sports group fosters camaraderie and offers the opportunity for bigger games and greater participation. Sport groups have generally received positive feedback, with the combined group being popular and a motivator for the clients to remain safe in order to be allowed to participate. A positive aspect has been the opportunity to build rapport with young people while they are participating in the sports group. The sports psychologist and exercise physiologist, when present, have provided coaching for the young people and mentorship for the group leaders. A limiting factor is poor participation by young people in the initial phase of their admission when they may be unable to engage for the whole hour owing to psycho-motor agitation or slowing. It is a challenge for the group leaders to come up with novel games for indoors that utilise the space creatively. Maintaining physical safety is also an important consideration. The psychologist and physiologist assisted greatly here with their expertise on technique. Fortunately to date there have been no major injuries, but cuts, bruises and sprains are relatively common. The standard procedure in the event of injury is to apply first aid and arrange review by a doctor. Warm ups and stretching are conducted prior to the activity to reduce the occurrence of such injuries without completely eliminating them. To prevent abscond-ing during outdoor activities risk assessments are conducted for each patient ahead of the activity. When doing an outdoor activity, a ratio of one staff to two patients is maintained to cover injury or absconding. Indoor activities are typically run by one staff member.

Another strategy to maintain healthy levels of physical activity is the daily supervised group walk on the grounds of the hospital. In summer months, this is augmented with the option of using the hospital swimming pool. When not restricted by COVID young people are offered a com-munity outing on alternate Friday afternoons. The outing usually involves physical activity, such as rock climbing or beach walking. Some young people have personalised fitness programmes, these days supervised by nursing staff who have a special interest in physical fitness. During unstruc-tured time, the young people are also encouraged to use the fitness equip-ment available in the courtyard areas. Consistently the most popular activity is the trampoline.

Analysis of patient data from 2015 to 2020 (n = 89) found a non-significant increase in mean BMI from admission to discharge of 25.45 to 25.70 (t = 0.67, p = 0.50). Aggregate data do not tell the full story, as some patients admitted to the Walker Unit were significantly underweight, while others were morbidly obese. Of those admitted with a BMI < 18 (n = 4), 100% gained weight. Of those admitted with a BMI > 30 (n = 18), 67% lost weight.

OTHER HEALTH PROBLEMS

Other than problems associated with overweight, accidental and self-inflicted injuries are the most common physical comorbidity experienced by the young people. Engagement in self-harm influences the young per-son's level (see Chap. 3). The threshold for determining if a young person will drop a level is if the self-injury required an intervention. Severity of self-injury ranges from minor to life-threatening. Hanging and ligaturing are generally the most serious events, and automatically trigger a call to the Medical Emergency Team (MET) based at the adjacent general hospital. Based on the MET assessment the young person is either managed conservatively on the Unit, or transferred to the general hospital for further assessment and management. A subcategory of self-harm is wound interference, where the young person picks at sutures or scar tissue to aggravate the wound. In such cases, we seek a consultation from the Plastic Surgery team. Sometimes the problem can be alleviated by placing a plaster cast over the wound, thus preventing access. Unfortunately, many young people find a way to wriggle out of the cast or to damage it so that they may again access their wound. In one case, a young person used her cast as a weapon against a staff member.

Infections and infestations occur occasionally, as they would anywhere young people are living together. The impacts of the COVID pandemic are described in Chap. 20. However, during the pandemic, the Unit has also had to deal with outbreaks of gastroenteritis and nits, both brought into the unit from home leave. In each case, management of the situation was well guided by infection control policy.

Of chronic medical comorbidities, seizure disorders and Type 1 diabetes are the most common. There is substantial planning prior to accepting patients with such conditions, to ensure that they can be managed safely. A weakness of the Walker Unit is its lack of proximity to paediatric services, which means that it is not possible for paediatricians to attend to provide consults. Instead, we have the more cumbersome arrangement of requesting outpatient consultations at the nearest children's hospital. Proximity to a paediatric unit would also have facilitated the rotation of paediatric nurses through the Walker Unit, a strategy which would have broadened our capacity to manage patients with significant medical comorbidity (Hazell, 2021). Fortunately, we have MET coverage from the adjacent general hospital, so that all urgent problems are addressed. Obtaining advice on longer term management can be a little more complicated.

Sleep problems are ubiquitous among young people referred to the Walker Unit. While we may maintain hypnotic medication initiated in the community in the short term, the focus shifts to improving sleep hygiene. The simple strategies of enforcing a quiet time before bed, stipulating a bedtime, and removing access to electronic devices after bedtime, coupled with an increase in daytime physical activity, is usually sufficient to overcome sleep phase delay and mid insomnia. Sleeping in is not permitted on school days. Young people with more entrenched sleep difficulties may be referred for a diagnostic sleep study.

Comorbid substance abuse affects only a minority of young people referred to the Walker Unit. Admission to the Unit significantly restricts the young person's capacity to access illicit substances, and the level of nursing observation makes it difficult for substance ingestion to go undetected. In recent times, only cigarettes and e-cigarettes have been detected on gown and room searches. Where there is suspicion a young person is using illicit substances while on leave, a urine sample will be obtained intermittently on their return to the Unit for the purposes of drug screening. Preventive education about substance misuse is provided in the Teenage Life group (see Chap. 9).

Acknowledgement Parisa Fani-Molky (medical student, The University of Sydney) assisted in the preparation of this chapter by retrieving data about patient BMIs.

REFERENCES

Carney, R. (2019). The 'obesogenic' environment of adolescent inpatient units: A call for action to support the promotion of better physical wellbeing. Retrieved September 27, 2021, from https://www.acamh.org/blog/obesogenic-adolescent-inpatient-units/

Carney, R., Imran, S., Law, H., Firth, J., & Parker, S. (2021). Physical health interventions on adolescent mental health inpatient units: A systematic review and call to action. *Early Interv Psychiatry, 15*(3), 439–448. https://doi.org/10.1111/eip.12981

Eapen, V., Faure-Brac, G., Ward, P. B., Hazell, P., Barton, G. R., Asghari, D., & P. (2012). Evaluation of weight gain and metabolic parameters among adolescent psychiatric inpatients: Role of health promotion and life style intervention programs. *Journal of Metabolic Syndrome, 1,* 109. https://doi.org/10.4172/2167-0943.1000109

Hazell, P. (2021). Debate: Inpatient units must enhance the system of care. *Child and Adolescent Mental Health, 26*(2), 176–177. https://doi.org/10.1111/camh.12459

CHAPTER 17

The Pharmacist and Pharmacotherapy

Jacky Hanh, Philip Hazell, and Isabelle Feijo

Abstract Clinical pharmacy services aim to optimise health outcomes and improve patient safety throughout all steps of the medicines management pathway, by ensuring the quality use of medicines and minimising medication-related problems. The role of the pharmacist includes gathering and documenting medication histories, performing medication reconciliation and undertaking clinical medication reviews. These services support collaborative approaches between patients, carers and the multidisciplinary team to develop patient-centred medication management plans. The practice of pharmacotherapy at the Walker Unit shares features in common with prescribing in acute child and adolescent mental health inpatient units, but there are some differences. This chapter will in particular seek to highlight the characteristics of pharmacotherapy that are distinct to longer stay intensive psychiatric care.

J. Hanh • I. Feijo
Walker Unit, Concord Centre for Mental Health, Concord, NSW, Australia
e-mail: Jacky.Hahn@health.nsw.gov.au; Isabelle.Feijo@health.nsw.gov.au

P. Hazell (✉)
Walker Unit, Concord Centre for Mental Health, Concord, NSW, Australia

The University of Sydney, Sydney, NSW, Australia
e-mail: Philip.Hazell@health.nsw.gov.au

© The Author(s) 2022
P. Hazell (ed.), *Longer-Term Psychiatric Inpatient Care for Adolescents*, https://doi.org/10.1007/978-981-19-1950-3_17

Keywords Adolescent • Inpatients • Mental health • Pharmacy service, Hospital • Medication therapy management

INTRODUCTION

Pharmacotherapy is the most common treatment used within mental health facilities with more than 90% of patients prescribed psychotropic medicines (Roughead et al., 2017). Due to their frequent use, they are associated with the highest incidence of errors and adverse events (Australian Commission on Safety and Quality in Health Care, 2017). It is believed that up to 50% of these incidences and adverse events are preventable (Australian Commission on Safety and Quality in Health Care, 2017). In 2019, the Australian Government declared quality use of medicines (QUM) and medicines safety as the tenth National Health Priority (Rigby, 2020). The basis of QUM and medicines safety is the judicious, appropriate, safe and efficacious use of all medicines (Rigby, 2020). The Medication Safety in Mental Health report published in 2017 by the Australian Commission on Safety and Quality in Health Care (ACSQHC) listed key recommendations to improve medicines safety within the mental health setting. The recommendations included adoption of clinical pharmacy services and medication reconciliation services (Roughead et al., 2017).

PHARMACY SERVICES

Clinical pharmacy services within the Walker Unit aim to optimise health outcomes and improve patient safety throughout all steps of the medication management pathway. The medication management pathway begins with the decision to prescribe a medicine, followed by the dispensing, administering and monitoring medicine use. Due to the complex and multidisciplinary nature of medication management, all stages of the medication management pathway can involve medication-related problems (MRPs) and adverse medication events. Pharmacists are well positioned to reduce these errors and adverse events, and evidence demonstrates that implementation of clinical pharmacy services results in improved and safer health care (Australian Commission on Safety and Quality in Health Care, 2017; Roughead et al., 2017). Key evidence-based services offered by pharmacists shown to improve patient outcomes include documentation of best possible medication histories (BPMH), performing medication reconciliation and undertaking clinical medication reviews. Pharmacists also provide clinical recommendations regarding therapeutic drug monitoring, drug interactions, management of adverse drug reactions, psychopharmacology as well as interpretation and application of pharmacogenomic testing. These services support a collaborative approach between patients, carers and the multidisciplinary team to develop patient-centred medication management plans.

Transition points of care are highly prone to unintended medication changes, with more than 50% of MRPs occurring at transitions of care and approximately 33% of these have the potential to cause harm (Australian Commission on Safety and Quality in Health Care, 2017). This is particularly true during hospital admissions due to the lack of accurate medication histories on presentation (Roughead et al., 2017). Some of the errors that can occur include unintentional discontinuation of therapy, recommencement of ceased medications, inappropriate orders and failure to identify MRPs. The Guide for Hospitals published by the National Safety and Quality Health Service Standards (NSQHSS) recommends that a BPMH is documented as soon as possible on admission to hospital. This BPMH should then be reconciled against the prescribed medication orders to correct any discrepancies. Documentation of a BPMH followed by reconciliation against the prescribed medication orders on admission has been shown to reduce medication errors by 50% to 94% (Australian Commission on Safety and Quality in Health Care, 2017).

Pharmacist-led documentation of BPMH and medication reconciliation are conducted for patients as soon as possible upon admission to the Walker Unit. The key steps in obtaining a BPMH involve obtaining two independent sources of medication lists and history of medication allergies and adverse drug events, with one source ideally being the patient or carer (Rigby, 2020). This BPMH is then documented in the patient's medication management plan on the electronic medical record to be accessible by the multidisciplinary team. The documented BPMH is then reconciled with the prescribed medication orders to identify and resolve MRPs and discrepancies such as omissions and duplications of therapy, and incorrect drug, dosages and frequencies. Similarly, the discharge transition point of care is also prone to unintended medication changes. Hence, a pharmacist-led discharge medication reconciliation process is also undertaken when patients are discharged from the Walker Unit. The discharge medication prescriptions are compared against the discharge plan and medication lists to ensure that changes are documented and unintended discrepancies are corrected.

Whilst documentation of BPMH and performing medication reconciliation greatly reduces MRPs, they have the greatest impact during transitions of care. On the other hand, well-structured clinical medication reviews ensure quality use of medicine (QUM) and medicines safety at all stages of the medication management pathway including when prescribing, dispensing and administering medications. Although clinical medication reviews are a multidisciplinary responsibility, the Society of Hospital Pharmacists of Australia indicates that pharmacists are expected to undertake clinical medication reviews within its Standards of Practice for Mental Health Pharmacy (Mahoney et al., 2009).

At the Walker Unit, pharmacist-led clinical medication reviews are conducted regularly for patients to detect and resolve MRPs, and to improve QUM and medication safety. These medication reviews include reviewing the current and newly prescribed medications, as well as previous medication use to optimise medication management. Outcomes of these medication reviews include clinical recommendations to improve therapeutic drug monitoring, management of drug interactions and adverse drug reactions, and advise on psychopharmacology and pharmacogenomics.

Therapeutic drug monitoring involves the measurement of drug concentration levels within bodily fluids to optimise efficacy, minimise toxicity and monitor adherence (Sansom, 2012). Therapeutic drug monitoring is employed for drugs with a narrow therapeutic index, defined therapeutic concentration range or established relationship between drug concentrations and clinical effect (Sansom, 2012). At the Walker Unit, medications that undergo therapeutic drug monitoring include lithium, valproate and clozapine. Monitoring and management of adverse drug reactions is an important role of mental health pharmacists. Over 80% of adult patients with psychotic illnesses experience some form of adverse drug reaction from their medications and approximately a third of these cause moderate to severe impairment (Roughead et al., 2017). Common adverse drug reactions handled by pharmacists at the Walker Unit include monitoring and management of metabolic side effects from antipsychotic use, as well as haematological and cardiovascular monitoring for clozapine patients. Management of adverse drug reactions may sometimes necessitate dosage reductions or cessation of therapy and the pharmacists are well situated to recommend strategies to avoid or minimise discontinuation syndromes.

With their expertise and training, pharmacists are also well equipped to improve QUM and medicines safety by providing advice on psychopharmacology. Pharmacists at the Walker Unit play a role in rationalisation of medication therapy, selection of medications, switching therapies and deprescribing. The increased accessibility of pharmacogenomic testing has provided mental health clinicians another tool to select the most appropriate medications for their patients particularly in cases of treatment resistance, or intense and unexpected adverse effects. Pharmacogenomic testing involves testing the genetic variances of a particular patient to better understand how they will respond to specific medications (Sansom, 2012). This allows for medication and dosage regimens to be individualised based on the patient's genetic makeup, thereby optimising a medication's effectiveness, and minimising the risk adverse reactions. However, the main challenges of utilising pharmacogenomics in the clinical setting are the training required to interpret genetic test results and the lack of guidelines on how to best modify therapy based on specific genetic variances (Sansom, 2012). Pharmacists are well equipped to overcome these challenges with their expertise in pharmacology and pharmacogenomics. They are also able to review the current literature to generate evidence-based recommendations on how to best individualise therapy based on genetic test results.

Additional clinical pharmacy services include facilitation of continuity of medication management through provision of updated medication lists as well as patient and carer medication counselling. Both activities align with the recommendations published by ACSQHC in their Guide for Hospitals. They recommend that health services should provide patients with sufficient information about their treatments and medications in a form appropriate to their level of health literacy (Australian Commission on Safety and Quality in Health Care, 2017). For these reasons, patients discharged from the Walker Unit are supplied an updated medication list and are counselled on their medication changes. The facility also offers its patients and carers access to the Choice and Medication website which provides a range of leaflets and fact cards on different mental illnesses and medications.

Pharmacotherapy

The practice of pharmacotherapy at the Walker Unit shares features in common with prescribing in acute child and adolescent mental health inpatient units, but there are some differences. For a start, if medication was the answer to a young person's difficulties they would not need the support of a longer stay unit. We therefore understate rather than overstate the likely benefits of medication. This section will in particular seek to highlight the characteristics of pharmacotherapy that are distinct to longer stay intensive psychiatric care.

Owing to the severity and chronicity of their problems, most young people on entry to the Walker Unit are prescribed a combination of medications. In addition, most young people will have previously had adequate or inadequate trials of many other psychotropic agents. Some will be experiencing impairing side effects. An important early task, usually delegated to the psychiatrist in training, is to develop a timeline of all previous treatment documenting where possible duration, maximum dose and perceived benefits or harms.

Unlike acute units, the Walker Unit is not under time pressure to rapidly initiate or alter treatment. Medication would only usually be amended at the point of admission if there was toxicity, risk to the physical health in the context of a severe psychotic or depressive illness or ongoing severe risk taking behaviour requiring regular sedation. Changes to treatment are made, if indicated, after several weeks of observation and diagnostic clarification. Medications are selected to target specific and problematic symptoms or diagnoses. Not every symptom or diagnosis requires a medication. Some are better addressed by non-pharmacological treatment; others do not require treatment at all. Where possible, the treatment is simplified. This is an important consideration for young people discharged to rural and remote areas where there is no access to paediatric psychopharmacology expertise

PRN (pro re nata or medication as needed) is a reality in an inpatient unit managing high risk and severely unwell patients. On admission, most patients are routinely charted the following to be administered for agitation or behavioural disturbance where other measures articulated in the 'de-escalation tree' (see Chap. 3) have been ineffective:

- lorazepam (oral)
- quetiapine (oral)

- midazolam (intramuscular)
- ziprasidone (intramuscular)

PRN medication may be modified according to the patient's circumstances and need. For example, in a patient routinely taking olanzapine, additional olanzapine may be preferable to administering quetiapine.

Especially for conditions relating to anxiety, depression and trauma the treatment emphasis is taken away from reliance on medication and redirected towards the importance of a healthy lifestyle including exercise and a balanced diet. Most patients have a one to two year history of slowly deteriorating illness, have not been attending school, socially isolating and been overly sedentary with unhealthy eating habits leading to unhealthy weight (too high or too low) which in return impacts their mental state.

In cases of early onset treatment resistant schizophrenia, some patients continue to deteriorate in their mental state despite being on therapeutic doses of clozapine or other antipsychotic medication. In these situations, time is taken to consider alterative medications and augmentation strategies leading to the least possible side effect profile. Parents may question the treatment and attribute the deterioration in mental state to the medication rather than the natural course of the illness. In these instances, psycho-education is of utmost importance to ensure the ongoing engagement of the family. In the most severe cases, it can take several months up to years before the illness stabilises and the patient can be discharged.

Conclusion

Thanks to the close collaboration on a weekly basis between the MDT and the pharmacist, the medication journey of the young person during their admission to the Walker Unit is optimised by reducing the side effect profile while increasing the efficacy of the medication regime. Every adjustment in medication is discussed with the young person and their family/carer to improve the compliance and awareness of the illness.

References

Australian Commission on Safety and Quality in Health Care. (2017). *National safety and quality health service standards guide for hospitals*. Commission on Safety and Quality in Health Care.

Mahoney, S., Zulli, A., & Walton, K. (2009). Patient satisfaction and energy intakes are enhanced by point of service meal provision. *Nutrition & Dietetics*, *66*(4), 212–220. https://doi.org/10.1111/j.1747-0080.2009.01373.x

Rigby, D. (2020). Medication reconciliation. *The Australian Journal of Pharmacy*, *101*(1196), 70–73.

Roughead, L. P. N., Westaway, K., Sluggett, J., & Alderman, C. (2017). *Medication safety in mental health*. Australian Commission on Safety and Quality in Health Care.

Sansom, L. (2012). *Australian pharmaceutical formulary and handbook* (22nd ed.). Pharmaceutical Society of Australia.

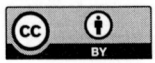

CHAPTER 18

The Policy Context and Governance

Beth Kotze

Abstract The Walker Unit opened in 2009 as the first of its kind in Australia to provide an intensive longer stay secure psychiatric inpatient rehabilitation programme for adolescents with severe mental illness who had not benefited from at least one but generally repeated admissions or prolonged care in other tertiary inpatient unit settings. Unusually, this happened at a time when the focus of reform in mental health at a State and National level is on community models, early intervention and community residential care rather than extended inpatient care in the specialist clinical sector. As a first of its kind, the Unit is an important innovation in inpatient mental health care and has garnered a reputation in the clinical sector for creating value in mental health care.

Keywords Adolescent • Inpatients • Mental health • Clinical governance • Benchmarking • Policy

B. Kotze (✉)
Child and Adolescent Mental Health Services, Sydney Local Health District, Sydney, NSW, Australia

Discipline of Psychiatry, The University of Sydney, Sydney, NSW, Australia

Faculty of Health, University of Technology, Sydney, NSW, Australia
e-mail: beth.kotze@health.nsw.gov.au

© The Author(s) 2022
P. Hazell (ed.), *Longer-Term Psychiatric Inpatient Care for Adolescents*, https://doi.org/10.1007/978-981-19-1950-3_18

DEVELOPING HIGHLY SPECIALIST SERVICES FOR SMALL
TARGET POPULATIONS

In NSW, Local Health Districts (LHDs) and Specialty Networks (SNs) have responsibility for planning of health services to meet local or defined population needs in consultation and jointly with the Ministry of Health and involving their local community (Health Services Act 1997 No 154). The Ministry of Health sets policy and strategic directions for the overall state health system and coordinates the planning and purchasing of system-wide services, including services across LHDs. In particular, the Ministry has a strong role in planning for highly specialised and low volume services that require a very specialised workforce for effective delivery. The Walker Unit is an example of a service that requires planning at the level of the population of the State because of the highly specialised nature of extended inpatient clinical mental health rehabilitation for adolescents and projected low volume.

The Ministry of Health planning process requires evidence of need and demand in a population for new services and evidence of effectiveness of interventions. An important development in Australia that leads this approach to mental health planning is the National Mental Health Services Planning Framework which was a commitment by the Australian Commonwealth Government under the Fourth National Mental Health Plan 2009–2014. This planning tool provides an 'internationally unprecedented, evidence-based framework providing national average benchmarks for optimal service delivery across the full spectrum of mental health services in Australia' (The University of Queensland, 2019). The Technical Appendices detail the complexity of development of the model in the face of available evidence and matching service elements to populations (The University of Queensland, 2016). Relevant insights are provided in the comments: 'The most critical data for estimating the impact of interventions are rarely available at all, let alone in a form useable for modelling' (page 16) and 'levels of demand may ... be invisible until a new service becomes available' (page 15). Hence, expert working groups were essential to establishing various elements of the model. This is demonstrated in a statement found in the section dealing with acute inpatient bed requirements for the 0–17 year old age group in the Service Element and Activity Descriptions (The University of Queensland, 2016). The section notes that 'Experts advised that beds may be arranged to provide collocated specialist sub-acute services for *small numbers of adolescents who may require extended stays'* (page 62; my emphasis). To plan specialist clinical rehabilitation inpatient services with extended stays for adolescents, one must look to the contemporary knowledge of specialists in the field.

The period 1996 onwards saw the expansion of acute child and adolescent mental health beds in NSW to the point of nine acute inpatient units networked across the state meeting the then population planning estimates to 2021. The planning for the Walker Unit was based on observations of small numbers of adolescents with severe complex and persistent mental illness for whom 'everything else' had been tried and who were 'stuck' in adult or adolescent acute beds. The general view was the care needs of this group overwhelmed the resources of specialist tertiary units, the stepdown from tertiary acute inpatient care to community care was too steep and the extended care needs of the group were ill-met in acute inpatient settings. Further, extended stays in child and adolescent acute mental health inpatient units were contributing to access block for acutely unwell adolescents and extended stays in adult inpatient units were developmentally inappropriate. The Walker Unit was planned as a supra-LHD service provided on behalf of the State to the population of NSW and the Australian Capital Territory at a time when no prototype for such highly specialised care existed in Australia.

IMPACT OF THE WALKER UNIT ON POLICY DEVELOPMENT

The Walker Unit is an example of how innovation in health is more often driven by service design than the traditional public policy model of policy cycles. Innovation is demonstrated in the way in which a customised solution was developed by experts for a significant problem impacting young people and their families and their illness trajectories leading to the proposal for a novel inclusion in the spectrum of child and adolescent mental health resources in NSW that would add value to the care provided for consumers and their families and the broader child and adolescent mental health service system.

At the time of the development of the Unit, the proposal that there would be value to the system was untested. It was a new idea that challenged assumptions that intensive community-based and acute inpatient care is 'enough' to meet the needs of this particular group of young people and the proposal involved considerable financial risk taking both in terms of capital and recurrent funding.

The Unit provides a specific and highly specialised inpatient rehabilitation service to NSW and Australian Capital Territory (ACT) for young people who are aged 12–18 years, have severe mental illness, have not benefited from care at a tertiary level and who are assessed as having potential to benefit from the extended secure care available at the Walker Unit. The provision of this level of child and adolescent mental health care would usually be associated with a Level 6 facility (the highest level in the NSW Role Delineation of Clinical Services 2019; note other elements of this classification level are not part of the facility from which the Walker Unit operates) and meets the NSW Health definition of a quaternary service in its meaning as an extension of tertiary care when the care is highly specialised and not widely accessed. The provision of such highly specialised services requires concentrated expertise and sufficient volume— meaning that there can realistically only be a small number or even one unit for a state, creating potential issues in access, continuity of care and vertical integration of specialised services and local specialist and primary care services.

This relates to another novel aspect to the Walker model—the Unit provides a discrete episode of care whilst actively working to maintain integration with local health and other service systems. One of the often-cited problems with a highly specialised child and adolescent mental health inpatient service is geographical dislocation for consumers and their families. This means that there are particular risks that can be anticipated and require mitigation, such as separation of young people from family and community supports; interrupted education, development and peer relationships; and, poor relational continuity of care that impacts on transitions to other forms of care. These risks are mitigated in the Walker model by several strategies. Firstly, the careful, comprehensive and collaborative assessment process that educates consumers, families/carers and referring agencies about what to expect. Secondly, the model ensures various ways, including but not limited to family therapy, of maintaining contact between the consumer and their family and ensuring that the parental role is not relinquished. Transitional planning is often complex and there may be many uncertainties during admission related to follow-up and stable accommodation in the community. Hence the model optimises available options including mobilising the support of the statutory child protection and education authorities to ensure maximum support and stability in follow-up.

GOVERNANCE AND POLICIES

Whilst the Ministry of Health has the role of coordinating the development and purchasing of supra-LHD services, the Local Health District from which the service is provided is responsible for service level monitoring consistent with local policies and procedures for Clinical Governance. This includes clinical care, adverse events and patient outcomes.

The Australian Commission on Safety and Quality in Health Care states 'Patient safety and quality systems are in place within governance processes to allow organisations to advance the safety and quality of patients' care' (Australian Commission on Safety and Quality in Health Care, 2017). The purpose of policies is to communicate values, philosophy and culture. Procedures on the other hand provide the process steps to follow and assign roles and responsibilities. The importance of these documents lies in promoting clear expectations, consistency, clarity and accountability and laying the groundwork for benchmarking, quality improvement, research and evaluation and generating evidence regarding best practice. This extends beyond, say, policies to deal with complaints to creative ways of engaging consumers and carers to bring their lived experience of care to influence all the various processes of care, challenging historical norms in practice and redesigning care towards what is valued highly by consumers and their families. The available evidence at this stage positively supports such consumer engagement to be important in outcomes of mental health care and successful transitional care.

In the case of the Walker Unit, the governance is within the context of a population-based mental health programme and ultimately within the context of an LHD, which is a statutory corporation, and the Board of the LHD. Formal structures and processes for reporting and policies and procedures provide a framework that supports a high level of decentralisation in clinical decision-making and policy implementation at the Unit level. Hence, the actual management of access of the population of NSW to the service is undertaken by the multidisciplinary team which allows for optimal processes of assessment, consent and engagement by consumers and families/carers and referring agents. Alternative methods such as centralised access management or collaborative governance with referring agents to manage access would be cumbersome and would not support this approach.

The philosophy of care integrates an understanding of the developmental stage of the adolescent and the stage of shared decision-making between the adolescent and their family/carers in addition to the severity and phase of illness. The model of care is strongly based in milieu therapies and psychosocial interventions in addition to family therapies, specialised psychological interventions and medical treatments. Physical health is a programme imperative and education is optimised. It is a complex model of care and the multiple components are tightly coupled. This is a strength of the model and supports the multidisciplinary team in being able to manage the ambiguity and complexity involved in the care of young people admitted to the Unit, including being able to manage issues like complex ethical dilemmas, including issues associated with use of the NSW Mental Health Act (2007) for involuntary care and child protection matters through multidisciplinary team processes. It also requires the team to critically review the model from time to time to ensure that it remains contemporary, best practice and evidence-based and continues to provide value to consumers and the system. The Unit has been subject to external peer review, participates in state-wide benchmarking and reports on its work and outcomes, such as in this publication. These clinical governance activities are all critical in demonstrating the value of the service.

However, the value approach to health care places emphasis on outcomes achieved against cost. To deliver value, a discrete episode of care is generally supported by optimal care pathways. To demonstrate value, evidence against the care pathways is required usually across the domains of outcomes, effectiveness and experience (of giving and receiving care). Such evidence is usually lacking in mental health yet is critical to the long-term sustainability of low volume highly specialised services. This publication positions the Unit well for the future by extending the work in the domain of value based health care, albeit a very complex undertaking.

Conclusion

The Walker Unit emerged over a decade ago as a novel idea developed by experts in response to a complex and significant gap in the care for young people with severe and persistent mental illness in NSW. A decade or more on and the leaders of the service are demonstrating the significant value of this service to a group of young people who are vulnerable to poor clinical outcomes with broad impact on their lives, their families and the community. The innovation established new policy and new perspectives on care for this group of consumers—the challenge now is to stay at the forefront of value by demonstrating outcomes against cost. This is challenging in the field of mental health. This book demonstrates how Walker programme is again innovating to meet this challenge.

REFERENCES

Australian Commission on Safety and Quality in Health Care. (2017). *National model clinical governance framework*. Sydney.

The University of Queensland. (2016). Technical Appendices for the Introduction to the National Mental Health Service Planning Framework—Commissioned by the Australian Government Department of Health. Version AUS V2.2. The University of Queensland, Brisbane.

The University of Queensland. (2019). Introduction to the national mental health service planning framework—Commissioned by the Australian Government Department of Health. Version AUS V2.2. The University of Queensland, Brisbane.

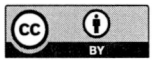

CHAPTER 19

Training and Education

Steve Hoare, Philip Hazell, Polly Kwan, Karen Sarmiento, and Bianca Lino

Abstract The Walker Unit has two principal educational functions; workforce development to increase the knowledge and skillset of clinicians, and supervised placement for students from a range of health disciplines. New appointees have access to an Introduction to CAMHS programme funded by the state government. The health service also provides orientation which incorporates mandatory training. In-house, the Walker Unit provides regular in-services to staff, and funds fortnightly supervision from an external provider. Advanced trainees in child and adolescent psychiatry and basic trainees in general psychiatry work in the unit. On observational placement are students from medicine, nursing, psychology, social work,

S. Hoare • P. Kwan • K. Sarmiento • B. Lino
Walker Unit, Concord Centre for Mental Health, Concord, NSW, Australia
e-mail: Steve.Hoare@health.nsw.gov.au; Polly.Kwan@health.nsw.gov.au; Karen.
Sarmiento@health.nsw.gov.au; Bianca.Lino@health.nsw.gov.au

P. Hazell (✉)
Walker Unit, Concord Centre for Mental Health, Concord, NSW, Australia

The University of Sydney, Sydney, NSW, Australia
e-mail: Philip.Hazell@health.nsw.gov.au

P. Hazell (ed.), *Longer-Term Psychiatric Inpatient Care for Adolescents*, https://doi.org/10.1007/978-981-19-1950-3_19

and occupational therapy. Attention is given to preparing students for the intense nature of the programme and the clinical environment.

Keywords Adolescent • Mental health • Staff development • Vocational education • Health education

INTRODUCTION

CAMHS inpatient units are well placed to provide vocational training in a range of mental health disciplines as they have an aggregation of skilled clinicians able to teach, and patients who are readily accessible. Early in his career, the editor of this e-textbook (PH) was surprised to visit a CAMHS inpatient unit that discouraged student placements, on the grounds that it disrupted patient care. In contrast, the team at the Walker Unit considers they have an obligation to support training and education to ensure there is a skilled workforce capable of delivering CAMHS inpatient care (Hazell, 2021). We aspire to make training placements available to all disciplines working within the unit, and to make placements available to people from outside of the local health district, including those who come from lower- and middle-income countries (Hazell, 2021).

GENERIC TRAINING

Staff newly appointed to the local health district receive one day of generic orientation to the health service. Nurses and midwives receive a further three days of discipline specific orientation. Topics covered are summarised in Box 19.1. To be frank, this is not the most thrilling experience for most inductees, but for a large organisation such as the Sydney Local Health District, it is a means to ensure all staff have received at least minimum exposure to knowledge essential to safe work practice.

Box 19.1 Topics covered during the generic orientation to the health service

Child protection
Domestic and family violence
Acceptable workplace behaviour (including The NSW Health Code of Conduct)
In-hospital emergencies
Fire and disaster management
Security and aggression
Environmental safety
Mask Fit Testing
Hazardous chemicals and substances
Manual handling
Safe work practices
Equipment safety
Incident and Injury Management System

Orientation is supplemented by further mandatory training that must be completed during the first year of employment (see Box 19.2). Some of the topics must be renewed annually. Completion of mandatory training is considered at each staff member's annual performance review.

Box 19.2 Generic mandatory training topics

Fire Training (Theory)*
Fire Training (Practical)*
Basic Life Support Assessment (Cardiopulmonary Resuscitation Practical)*
Basic Life Support—Adult (Online Theory)*
Hand Hygiene
Infection Prevention and Control Practices (for clinical staff)
Mental Health Clinical Handover
Working with consumers and communities

(continued)

(continued)
Violence Prevention and Management—Personal Safety
Child Wellbeing and Child Protection
Introduction to Safety and Quality
Detecting Deterioration, Evaluation, Treatment, Escalation and Communicating in Teams
Introduction to Work, Health, and Safety
Open Disclosure
Privacy
Care Coordination
*renewed annually

CAMHS Training (external)

Within two years of commencing in their first position in a child and adolescent mental health service, staff may also undertake a four day introductory course under the auspices of the NSW Ministry of Health (see Box 19.3). The training is informed by the NSW Child and Adolescent Mental Health Services (CAMHS) Competency Framework (NSW Ministry of Health, 2011). In addition, the NSW Ministry of Health provides scholarships for staff to undertake more intensive study in child and adolescent mental health through courses offered by the Health Education and Training Institute (Health Education and Training Institute, 2021), summarised in Box 19.4.

Box 19.3   Topics covered in the Introduction to CAMHS course

Engagement, assessment, formulation, and developmentally appropriate interventions
   Working with culturally diverse communities
   Common mental health presentations that affect children and young people
   Evidence based interventions, including CBT, family therapy, and mindfulness.

Box 19.4   Topics covered in the HETI Graduate Certificate in Child and Youth Mental Health

Mental Health, Mental Ill Health, and Suicide
Strength-Based Assessment and Care Planning
Professional and Ethical Mental Health Care
Attachment Development and Promoting Mental Health Across the Lifespan
Sustaining your mental health practice
Core Therapeutic Skills
Child and Youth Mental Health Conditions 1
Child and Youth Mental Health Conditions 2
Diversity and Mental Health
Child and Youth Mental Health Conditions 3
Trauma-Informed Care and Practice **or** Recovery and Recovery-Oriented Practice
Legal and Ethical considerations for Child and Youth Mental Health

GENERAL WORKPLACE TRAINING

Generic training has a role, but staff working at the Walker Unit require more specific in-house training and supervision to enable them to perform their roles. All staff are invited to participate in bi-weekly sessions with an external supervisor, although in practice the session is mostly attended by allied health and medical staff. The focus may be a particular case, or it may be an issue that is of concern to the multidisciplinary team. Examples of the latter include reflection on the suicide death of a former patient, adjustment to COVID related restrictions in practice, and the right of young people under the age of 16 to exclude certain family members from their family therapy. Sessions are documented by the team and by the supervisor. We find this helpful as it enables us to identify recurring themes. Discipline specific supervision is also available for most professions. There have been challenges accessing people with sufficient relevant experience to supervise occupational therapy, speech pathology, and art therapy.

We hold ad hoc staff development sessions on topics of salience to the unit. Recent topics include the use of structured diagnostic interviews, the role of art therapy, collaborative care planning, and the manner of conducting a gown search for high risk patients returning from leave.

DISCIPLINE SPECIFIC TRAINING

Nursing

The Walker Unit hosts nursing staff new to mental health undertaking their one year "Transition to Mental Health Nursing" course for a three month rotational placement. Allocation to a CAMHS unit can be requested by staff if preferred but is typically allocated based on staffing requirement within the service. The transition to mental health nursing course does not of itself offer any specific CAMHS training, beyond an introductory lecture that describes the health districts services for young people and their families. When assigned to the Walker Unit, transition nurses are allocated two preceptors from the established staff to support their orientation and participation into the ward activities. In addition to the one day personal safety training, all nursing staff are required to complete a three day course in violence prevention and management so that they can form part of the service duress response teams. For staff who identify CAMHS as their preferred work environment, enrolment in the Introduction to CAMHS course already mentioned is undertaken within their first two years. For more advanced clinicians, consideration to undertake CAMHS related courses is done on an individual basis, but it includes courses facilitated by the Health Education Training Institute described in Box 19.4. The unit has monthly group clinical supervision for nursing staff conducted by an external Clinical Nurse Consultant who reflects upon situations identified by the group of staff attending during the meeting. Another form of reflective practice is undertaken in monthly Incident Review Meetings, which is part of a wider mental health service initiative to learn from incidents and reflect on practice.

Nursing student placements vary in length, typically between two and four weeks in duration. Students are directly supported by a clinical facilitator from their university, and ordinarily are exposed to a range of activities common among the whole mental health service; visiting the ECT clinic, observing a mental health tribunal being conducted and participating in debriefs among their cohort to reflect upon their experiences.

Nursing students are allocated a registered nurse to shadow on a shift by shift basis, whom share and supervise students conducting day to day activities. At the Walker Unit, the emphasis for nursing students is both safe engagement with young people and attendance at the weekly case review, to observe how decisions in care are made by the whole multidisciplinary team. Nursing staff supervising students have access to an array of CAMHS specific literature to provide students and assist them in their learning experience.

Psychiatry

Psychiatrists in training work in the unit. Most are completing their six month compulsory term in child and adolescent psychiatry, which is usually undertaken in Stage 2 of the RANZCP training programme. Less commonly, we have an advanced trainee in child and adolescent psychiatry (Stage 3 of RANZCP training) who will be completing a compulsory inpatient term. The term offers the psychiatrists in training exposure to severe and complex psychopathology, and intensive therapeutic work. However, we have to arrange experiences offsite to ensure the Stage 2 trainees have the necessary exposure to children under 13 years of age, and become familiar with high prevalence, mild to moderate severity conditions. We achieve this through clinic sessions in community CAMHS and consultation to community child health clinics. Because the consultant psychiatrists in the unit are 'hands on' with their clinical care and the allied health and nursing staff are very capable, there is a danger that psychiatrists in training are supernumerary to the programme. We try to overcome this by ensuring the psychiatrists in training have specific tasks (e.g. preparing the documentation required to present a patient to the Mental Health Tribunal) and that they are allocated therapeutic roles such as being a patient's individual psychotherapist. In addition to the psychiatrists in training, we support observerships for psychiatry residents from other countries. To date we have hosted psychiatry residents from Asia, South America, and Southern Europe. Such observerships typically last three months. The resident participates in most ward activities, but is not authorised to treat patients.

Psychology

Provisional psychologists undertake supervised placements in the unit of up to six months, on a part-time basis. Most of these students are completing the placement as part of an APAC (Australian Psychology Accreditation Council)-accredited higher education programme (Masters or Doctorate in Clinical Psychology). The students have an opportunity to contribute to all parts of the Walker programme, including, individual therapy, group therapy, multidisciplinary team meetings and team supervision, and do so under the guidance of experienced clinical psychologists. Owing to the severe and complex nature of the presentations of patients at the Walker Unit, students are interviewed before being offered a position and the positions are typically offered to students as a final placement prior to entering the workforce, or to students who have prior experience with similar patient populations.

Social Work

The health district's Mental Health Social Work and Psychology Educator coordinates all field placements and provides support for both the student and supervisor for the duration of the placement. To support each student's integration into placement the Educator provides a comprehensive orientation to the service at the beginning of placement to all social work and psychology students. Ongoing learning is fostered through fortnightly education sessions in the areas of vicarious trauma, simulated learning, the National Disability Insurance Scheme, and its interface with mental health services, working with psychosis, sexual assault, family violence, alcohol and other drugs, and the justice system and mental health. The Educator also provides social work- specific fortnightly group supervision sessions to support students with any placement issues as well as to introduce key therapeutic tools utilised within general social work practice including: genograms, Eco maps, Theory circle, process recording and critical reflection. This is in addition to weekly individual clinical supervision provided by the placement supervisor.

Occupational Therapy

Occupational therapy fieldwork placement at the Walker Unit is offered to students in their third year of study or above. Students provide a brief description of their previous clinical experience and their learning goals prior to commencement. The placements are typically full time, with a duration of seven to ten weeks. Occupational therapy students are a great asset to the unit as they are expected to take on individual case loads and facilitate in the group therapy programme under supervision.

Medical Students

Students from The University of Sydney typically may spend two weeks attached to the unit during their Psychiatry and Addictions Medicine term. The placement is not mandatory, so most students who attend have specifically requested some exposure to child and adolescent psychiatry. All students, however, have access to online lectures and a case-based tutorial. For students seeking more extensive experience in child and adolescent psychiatry, we offer a personalised pathway programme which involves regular association with the Unit for up to a year. Additionally, medical students from Sydney and other universities may undertake an intensive elective placement, usually full time for four weeks.

Student Wellbeing

We stress to students attending the Unit that what they see is not representative of child and adolescent psychiatry in general. The patients we manage are severely impaired, and their problems are enduring. Intervention is delivered at a much greater intensity than one might see in a community setting, or in an acute inpatient unit. The general principles of our approach do, however, generalise to other treatment settings. We are mindful that some of the things students observe or hear about will be confronting to them. Examples include the disfigurement caused by self-mutilation, and bizarre body movements associated with neuropsychiatric disorder. As far as possible we prepare students, and are available to debrief them following exposure. Student safety is also a paramount concern. Students have not generally undertaken the extensive orientation and mandatory training required of paid staff. In addition, they do not have the clinical experience necessary to recognise when there is an escalating risk of aggression. As such, all student contacts with patients are supervised by an experienced member of staff.

REFERENCES

Hazell, P. (2021). Debate: Inpatient units must enhance the system of care. *Child and Adolescent Mental Health, 26*(2), 176–177. https://doi.org/10.1111/camh.12459

Health Education and Training Institute. (2021). Child and youth mental health services scholarship. Retrieved October 11, 2021, from https://www.heti.nsw.gov.au/Placements-Scholarships-Grants/scholarships-and-grants/child-and-adolescent-mental-health-services

NSW Ministry of Health. (2011). *NSW child and adolescent mental health services (CAMHS) competency framework.* NSW Ministry of Health, Sydney.

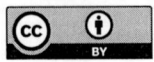

CHAPTER 20

Postscript: Responding to the COVID-19 Pandemic

Stephen Ho, Isabelle Feijo, and Philip Hazell

Abstract The risk posed to health facilities by COVID-19 is well recognised. From the first wave of infections in 2020, protective measures have been in place. In accordance with health district policy, staff and visitors were screened before entry to the Walker Unit. Along with the rest of the world, Walker staff became familiar with conducting meetings through online platforms such as Zoom. Compliance with ever changing infection control directives was a challenge, indeed a threat to the viability of the programme. There have been direct impacts on the operation of the Walker Unit, with travel and visiting severely restricted. The chapter will outline the adaptations made to the Walker programme through the pandemic.

S. Ho • I. Feijo
Walker Unit, Concord Centre for Mental Health, Concord, NSW, Australia
e-mail: Stephen.Ho@health.nsw.gov.au; Isabelle.Feijo@health.nsw.gov.au

P. Hazell (✉)
Walker Unit, Concord Centre for Mental Health, Concord, NSW, Australia

The University of Sydney, Sydney, NSW, Australia
e-mail: Philip.Hazell@health.nsw.gov.au

P. Hazell (ed.), *Longer-Term Psychiatric Inpatient Care for Adolescents*, https://doi.org/10.1007/978-981-19-1950-3_20

Keywords COVID-19 • Inpatients • Personal protective equipment • Infection control

INTRODUCTION

Rates of psychiatric morbidity among young people have risen in most countries during the course of the COVID-19 pandemic (Organisation for Economic Co-operation and Development, 2021). At the same time, mental health services and support for young people have been heavily disrupted by the COVID-19 crisis. A World Health Organisation survey in June-August 2020 found that in more than three-quarters of countries globally school mental health programmes were completely or partially disrupted, while in over 70% of countries child and adolescent mental health services experienced disruptions (World Health Organisation, 2020). At the time of writing, data about the effect on demand for and delivery of specialist inpatient mental health services for young people are limited. One acute adolescent inpatient service in the United States reported a reduction in the number of referrals, but a modest increase in length of stay. Of diagnoses at admission, there was a significant increase only in substance use disorder (Ugueto & Zeni, 2021). Owing to the quaternary nature of the service delivered by the Walker Unit we did not anticipate, and have not observed, a change in the pattern of referrals to us. Adjustments required by the pandemic have, however, had a substantial impact on the service we provide.

The Walker Unit, like the rest of the Health Service, has undergone significant change with periods of increased restriction that have intensified with each subsequent outbreak of the disease. The Unit has applied successfully for exemption from some directives, such as the prohibition of consumer leave. We argued that consumer leave was an essential component of progression towards discharge (see Chap. 4). As the service devised standard operating procedures (SOPs) subject to reviews, constant updates based on the latest health advice from the ministry, we provided input into what could be implemented. It took some time for staff, patients and families to adjust to each rule change. We soon realised that clear communication, co-operation and compassion promoted compliance.

WARD STRUCTURE

Following the first COVID-19 outbreak in Australia in March 2020 the hospital management visited every ward to decide where suspected and confirmed cases would be isolated. The Unit Director and Nurse Unit Manager (NUM) were consulted about balancing patients' needs against compliance with COVID-19 screening requirements. Following consultation, we identified two quarantine areas in the ward. Initially we designated one bedroom as the 'COVID bedroom' as well as the seclusion area as containment area as a last resort for uncooperative patients. Isolating young people in a designated bedroom without access to their parents and interacting only with fully 'gowned up' staff members was at times challenging. We reduced the stress by facilitating frequent contact with family members over phone or Facetime. On one occasion, a young person exited the bedroom and potentially infected the whole corridor. They threatened staff with a sharp object requiring police intervention and relocation of the young person to the seclusion room where they were nursed until the COVID test result came back negative.

It became clear to us that a single bedroom without an en-suite was an unsatisfactory quarantine area, so we switched this function to the bedroom located in the Pod area once it became available (see Chap. 2).

PERSONAL PROTECTIVE EQUIPMENT

In line with CEC recommendations and NSW Health Directive, from the first lockdown, staff and visitors were required to wear surgical masks in all clinical areas. All staff received training in the donning and doffing of personal protective equipment (PPE). When there was a suspected COVID-19 case, any staff member approaching the young person was required to wear PPE. Depending on the different levels of alert (green, amber or red) we were required to use face masks in only the clinical areas or in all areas of the Unit. In July 2021 we entered for the first time the red alert level which required the use of plastic goggles or shield (if wearing glasses) to protect from droplet transmission to the eyes. Seeing staff wearing PPE drew various reactions from the young people. There was a mix of curiosity, fear and confusion. We tried to mitigate patient anxiety through updates about COVID related matters at the community meeting. Eventually, seeing staff wearing masks and PPE became the 'new normal' for the young people.

Admission Planning

The first step of admission planning comprises an assessment of the young person and their family at the location where they are admitted or followed up (e.g. outpatient CAMHS) (see Chap. 4). During the initial outbreak of COVID-19, we transitioned to virtual meetings using the Zoom platform to assess the patient and their family. Unfortunately, the connection was intermittently unstable rendering the picture and sound quality poor. We found it difficult to get an accurate impression of the young person and their family, and engagement with the family was compromised. Overall, we found that for a sensitive process such as engagement and assessment, virtual technology was a poor substitute for meeting face to face. Whenever restrictions were relaxed, we have reverted to face to face assessments. The second step consists of the pre-admission meeting visit to the Walker Unit (see Chap. 4). We have continued to insist that the young person and family visit the unit in person, while observing infection control measures. On one occasion, we trialled a virtual tour of the ward, but found this method poorly suited to purpose.

The third step is the actual admission. Our procedure is to invite one parent to come to the Unit to help to settle the young person into the new milieu. We maintained this throughout the COVID-19 outbreak to reduce the stress linked to a transfer from another hospital or an admission from the community.

Staff Meetings

The hospital administration enforced a limit on the number of people who could be in the same room, based on a rule of four square metres per person. We had to rethink how to organise routine meetings such as morning handover, the case review and supervision. We transitioned to hybrid meetings, with some staff attending in person while others attended virtually using the Zoom platform. An unintended benefit was that hospital administration invested in better quality laptop computers for our staff, and upgraded the sound system in the main meeting room. In addition, staff could join meetings even if they were offsite. This was of great benefit on occasions when individuals were required to isolate at home.

School Programme

During the first lockdown, the Department of Education decided to remove the teaching staff from face to face teaching and change to online learning. As most of the young people at the Walker Unit have a long history of not attending school for various reasons, it was very difficult to maintain a structure. The allied health and nursing team 'stepped up' and we had rotations of different allied health members and nursing staff supporting both learning centres for two learning periods from Mondays to Fridays. After the restrictions were eased, the teaching staff was allowed back on the ward. Lessons learned from the first wave of the pandemic led to a different approach when the second wave again caused school closures. Our school principal advocated for a continuation of face to face teaching. To enable this some adaptations were required, such as using the dining room as main classroom and requiring the students to wear surgical masks. The now multipurpose area was regularly cleaned and disinfected. Another challenge arising from school lockdowns was disruption to the school re-integration process (see Chap. 7). As such, some young people were discharged without a successful re-integration, while for others discharge was delayed.

Group Programme

The Walker Unit followed the MHS advice on a risk-based approach to managing groups during the pandemic. This included identifying hazards and controls to manage COVID-19. The group facilitators took on the marshalling role, environmental management, ensuring compliance with social distancing and hand hygiene practices being followed as well as recording details of the group times and size limits to conform to the recommended limit of no longer than one hour per session.

During the outbreak in March 2020, we were restricted to no more than three students per group. To maintain continuity of the group therapy programme two small groups were run in parallel, switching over after half an hour. This was obviously much more labour intensive and not sustainable in the longer term. The other imposed restriction was that the young people were not allowed to go on group outings which made them feel even more restricted. These adaptations were similar to those reported from acute inpatient settings (Leffler et al., 2021). As an alternative to outings, we used the courtyards as often as possible to provide the young people with exposure to fresh air and sunlight. As soon as the restrictions eased after the first wave of the pandemic daily walks were reinstated. During the second wave, walks were permitted. Outings, however, have been subject to the community restrictions in force at any given time.

INDIVIDUAL THERAPY

Each patient is allocated an individual therapist for the duration of the admission (see Chap. 10). The pandemic has had less impact on individual therapy than other treatment modalities. For some patients Exposure and Response Prevention (ERP) therapy is indicated. ERP is usually undertaken in the community but the pandemic restrictions have required us to deliver ERP on the ward.

FAMILY THERAPY

Family therapy had to be modified during the initial outbreak. We continued to see all family members in person in the first month of admission as this is the time where we connect with the family and work on the Genogram and timeline. After this initial phase we would see one or both parents in person and have other family members over Zoom or phone conference. During the second outbreak, we had the Pod area available for family sessions. Families could access this part of the facility without coming through the ward area, which was of benefit in reducing the risk of contamination. After each use, the Pod was cleaned and disinfected.

As leave with family and to the family home is an important part of the therapy process, we continued to grant leave with the precaution of families being asked not to go to any public place during the leave period in order to diminish the risk of contamination. Complications did occur when young people absconded during their leave, or self-harmed requiring attendance at their local Emergency Department. In such cases, we isolated the patient on their return to the ward until they received a negative COVID test.

MORALE

The experience of the pandemic has challenged staff morale. It is disappointing not to be able to provide the full range and quality of clinical service the Walker programme has to offer. There is an ever present threat that a positive COVID-19 case among patients or staff could lead to ward closure. Constant changes in advice and procedures have been frustrating. But we are fortunate that most staff have been able to continue in their substantive clinical roles. Staff absences owing to the need for isolation have been minor. However, there remains a threat to the workforce when restrictions ease and the numbers of COVID-19 cases are predicted to rise. Informal staff interaction (e.g. staff farewells, social and morale boosting gatherings) has been restricted, but not completely eliminated. One project that has served to encourage staff unity has been the writing of this textbook.

CONCLUSION

The Walker team was able to continue to deliver treatment to the most vulnerable and unwell young people of the state of NSW throughout the COVID-19 epidemic and despite having had many suspected positive COVID cases, to the date of when this e-book was written we have not had any confirmed COVID cases within the patient population or the Walker Unit staff (including education department staff).

PPS

Just as the manuscript was being finalised for submission, a student nurse on placement at the Walker Unit tested positive for COVID. Within weeks several staff and patients contracted the illness. Young people who fell ill while on leave were granted extended leave to isolate at home. Those who developed symptoms while on the ward were isolated from the other patients. For a period the unit was in lockdown, with no visitation and no leave privileges.

REFERENCES

Leffler, J. M., Esposito, C. L., Frazier, E. A., Patriquin, M. A., Reiman, M. K., Thompson, A. D., & Waitz, C. (2021). Crisis preparedness in acute and intensive treatment settings: Lessons learned From a year of COVID-19. *Journal of the American Academy of Child and Adolescent Psychiatry, 60*(10), 1171–1175. https://doi.org/10.1016/j.jaac.2021.06.016

Organisation for Economic Co-operation and Development. (2021). Supporting young people's mental health through the COVID-19 crisis. Retrieved September 21, 2021, from https://www.oecd.org/coronavirus/policy-responses/supporting-young-people-s-mental-health-through-the-covid-19-crisis-84e143e5/

Ugueto, A. M., & Zeni, C. P. (2021). Patterns of youth inpatient psychiatric admissions before and after the onset of the COVID-19 pandemic. *Journal of the American Academy of Child and Adolescent Psychiatry, 60*(7), 796–798. https://doi.org/10.1016/j.jaac.2021.02.006

World Health Organisation. (2020). The impact of COVID-19 on mental, neurological and substance use services.

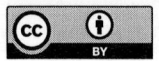

Correction to: Art Therapy

Fran Nielsen

CORRECTION TO:

Chapter 11 in: P. Hazell (ed.), *Longer-Term Psychiatric Inpatient Care for Adolescents*, https://doi.org/10.1007/978-981-19-1950-3_11

The book was inadvertently published with an error: There is a misplaced reference to image 11.5 in the book version of PDF and Chapter 11, which has been corrected.

The updated version of the chapter can be found at
https://doi.org/10.1007/978-981-19-1950-3_11

C2

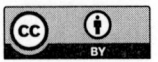

INDEX

© The Author(s) 2022
P. Hazell (ed.), *Longer-Term Psychiatric Inpatient Care for
Adolescents*, https://doi.org/10.1007/978-981-19-1950-3